Curing Cancer
with Carrots

Ann Cameron

Also available for Amazon Kindle and Barnes and Noble Nook e-readers and apps.

ISBN: 0692521763
ISBN-13: 978-0692521762 (Ann Cameron Books)

To Geoff, and in Memory of Bill

Table of Contents

Introduction   1
One: How the Numbers Melted   4
Two: A Letter and a Phone Call   16
Three: The Shooter Misses   21
Four: Falcarinol and Luteolin   28
Five: Juicing Carrots   31
Six: Treating the Community of Cells   41
Seven: Apoptosis and Necrosis   50
Eight: Caution and Chemotherapy   55
Nine: Carrot Liberation   61
Ten: Puzzles of Profitability   65
Eleven: Making Decisions   70
Twelve: Cures and Improvements   89
The Future?   101
Notes   102

The day is coming when
a single carrot
freshly observed
will set off
a revolution.

— Paul Cezanne (1839-1906)

Introduction

I'm the author of many children's books—stories in which adventurous children use their imaginations to solve problems in their lives. Mostly my books are funny and have happy endings. I never aspired to write a book about cancer. Cancer is not funny. Many of my friends found no solution for it. Slowly or fast, it killed them.

Then I got cancer. A few friends started sounding strange in a kindly way—as people do when they have decided you're about to die, but believe you haven't realized it yet.

I had surgery for the initial cancer and hoped I was okay. When I learned the cancer had metastasized, I too thought I had a death sentence. The surgeon told me I had two or three years to live. Amazingly, the metastasis disappeared quickly. I had no chemotherapy or radiation. The only change I made in my life was to drink five glasses of fresh carrot juice every day.

Seven weeks after I began the carrot treatment, a CT scan showed the cancer arrested, and the two tumors between my lungs shrinking. In nine more weeks another CT scan showed no tumors. I felt great. Joint and muscle pain that had been bothering me also disappeared; and my mood was excellent.

I cured my cancer using only carrots. This may sound like a fairy tale; many people can't understand how such a gentle cancer cure can work. The explanation comes from new findings in the field of nutritional epigenetics—the study of how hundreds of specific compounds in our diet affect the expression of our genes, turning off or turning on those that suppress or promote cancer.

Despite the wealth of scientific studies in this field, physicians, just like the rest of us, are often unaware of them. These studies could—and most certainly should—revolutionize the treatment of cancer, reducing the fear, suffering and cost of treatment. By learning about them you may be able to save yourself from cancer.

Centuries ago, rickets and scurvy were incurable scourges of humanity. Then we learned they were diseases of malnutrition. Cancer researchers believe that dietary changes could prevent up to two thirds of all cancers.[1] No matter what originally sparks cancer, in many cases it takes hold and grows because of nutritional deficiencies.[2] Once people get cancer, 80% of them suffer malnutrition caused as much by chemotherapy and radiation as by the disease itself.

In the not-so-distant past, doctors applied leeches to patients' bodies for bloodletting, cleaned wounds with mercury, and delivered babies with dirty hands. I believe the day will come when treatment of cancer by radiation and chemotherapy will be equally obsolete. Cancer will be prevented and in many cases, cured painlessly through specific nutritional changes.

Nearly one out of four Americans dies from cancer. Only five to ten percent of these cancers are genetic.[3] 10% are caused by lack of exercise; 30% are caused by smoking; 30-35% are caused by obesity, or diets with too much meat, fat and sugar, and not enough fruits and vegetables. These cancers are preventable. We can take responsibility for the way we live and stop them before they happen.[4] If we do get cancer, we can cure it. I did it. You and those you love can do it, too.

Curing Cancer with Carrots is my contribution to awareness about curing cancer with natural means. It's based on research from dozens of scientific journals. It explains how to juice carrots and presents new and exciting evidence of their cancer-curing effects. Apart from its focus on carrots, it's a useful, concise and clear guide for anyone dealing with cancer. It can help cancer patients and their families evaluate their situations and understand oncologists' language. It could prevent long hospitalizations and bankruptcy caused by medical treatment. It can show you how to take responsibility for your own health, do your own research, and make informed decisions. It just might save your life.

One: How the Numbers Melted

Only now that I am free of cancer am I beginning to recognize how scared I was in my journey through it. My doctors and nurses urged me to be brave and take on the pains and risks of chemotherapy. I didn't. Sometimes, fear is a virtue! I was worried about chemo's effects—its so-called "side" effects, which are often much more powerful than the intended effects of these drugs. My fears pushed me to think for myself and do my own research.

My cancer adventure started innocuously.

In August of 2011, I didn't have much energy. I figured that was normal, the result of ageing—just the way people feel when they're over sixty-five. Even so, I mentioned my lethargy to the nurse practitioner at the small Portland, Oregon clinic where I got my medical care. The nurse ordered a blood test. When it showed I was anemic, she prescribed iron pills. The iron pills didn't work. The other nurse in the practice prescribed more iron pills. Neither of them told me that anemia in older people is almost always a sign of internal bleeding, and that colon cancer is often its source.

Standard medical practice is to send anemic patients over age 60 for colonoscopies.[1] The nurses didn't order or even suggest a colonoscopy to me. They encouraged me to exercise more. I kept taking iron pills and became less anemic. But there were other signs that I wasn't well. In October 2011, a respiratory infection shook my whole body with coughing, so much so that I had to cancel a publishing trip I was on. The infection lasted for over a month. I'd never been that sick with a cold before. In December 2011, I went to a gym, where a young trainer urged me to hold a "plank" position on my elbows and toes for a minute. I did that a number of times over the course of a few weeks. Afterward I felt pain in my abdomen sporadically. I was sure I'd strained a muscle doing the plank. Friends suggested that having a young trainer who might overestimate one's strength is a bad idea. Better to join a gym that only has members over age fifty, they said. There was no such gym near me. I just gave up going to the one I'd joined.

I figured the muscle strain would improve eventually. I never mentioned it at the clinic. I didn't know that anemia and abdominal pain are the classic signs of colon cancer.

I live part of the year in Guatemala. I returned there in January 2012. In February, I took a boat trip on beautiful Lake Atitlán in the highlands. The waves were high. The boat slammed and bounced against them. I felt acute pain in my abdomen. At the end of February 2012, I saw a trauma specialist in Guatemala City. I explained that because of exercises I'd done in December, plus the punishing boat trip, I had a muscle problem—lots of abdominal pain. The specialist ordered an ultrasound. The radiologist reported that I had a lot of gallstones, but that my abdomen was normal. It turns out that an ultrasound doesn't provide the clear images needed to detect abdominal cancer. A CT is needed. I didn't know that.

I didn't know either, that confidently explaining to a doctor what is wrong with you may prevent him or her from arriving at a proper diagnosis. A friend saw the same Guatemala City specialist shortly before I did. She told him she had mysterious pains in her abdomen and had no idea why. For her, he ordered a CT. (Luckily, she was fine.)

When I returned to Portland in March, I brought with me two intestinal infections. The doctor at the Portland clinic didn't notice one of them on the lab report, so she didn't treat it. ("There was a lot of information on the report," she explained, apologizing.) I didn't see the report myself. Now I think anyone who sees a doctor should get copies of all lab reports. I didn't know that.

In March, my right abdomen hurt so much when I lay down on a bed that I had to do it very carefully to avoid acute pain. In April, the pain in my abdomen became a continuous dull ache, which I attributed to the intestinal infections. I couldn't go anywhere because of the diarrhea. I was more anemic than ever and very weak. I lay in bed day after day hoping the third and fourth round of powerful antibiotics kicking me in the gut would conquer the intestinal infection. Finally, I realized I needed a better doctor.

I went to a large clinic connected with Legacy Good Samaritan Hospital in Portland, where a new primary care doctor looked up the old lab report on his computer, and noticed the second intestinal infection. He prescribed an even stronger and more horrible medicine than the previous antibiotics. But in two weeks, it cured the infection.

It was early May. I expected to start feeling good again; but instead, my right abdomen, which had been tender and painful now felt entirely rigid. It felt as if the rigid area had doubled in size in a week. I went back to my new doctor and told him that curing the bacterial infection hadn't fixed my health. The abdominal pain I had attributed to a few exercises I'd done in December was still with me, only worse. He sent me for a CT scan. It showed a mass in my abdomen, probably colon cancer. He referred me to a surgeon. The surgeon rearranged his schedule to operate on me four days later, on June 9. He gave me a blood transfusion so I could withstand the five-hour operation and removed 12 inches of my colon, some lymph nodes, and a palm-sized area of muscle in my right abdomen.

He was jubilant over the success of the surgery. The removed lymph nodes weren't cancerous and their margins were clear, he said. Much later, he mentioned that if I had had surgery back in August 2011 when the first lab report showed I was anemic, he wouldn't have had to remove my abdominal muscles. Unfortunately, abdominal muscles, once gone, don't grow back.

In the first weeks after surgery, all that mattered to me was that he had saved my life. I hoped my cancer ordeal was over; but he said that, although chemotherapy was "controversial in my case" and "not mandatory," he recommended it. His words clearly suggested that for my case, other authorities *didn't* recommend chemo; but I didn't ask him to explain why not. When one's life is at stake it's worth hearing all points of view about a proposed treatment, but I didn't do it. I trusted him and accepted his referral to an oncologist.

For me, the very word "oncologist" rang with deathly overtones, but my new doctor was cheerful, easy to talk to and obviously knew her business. She didn't seem to belong in such a grim profession. I asked her why she hadn't chosen a happier specialty than oncology—maybe sports medicine? She told me firmly that she didn't like sports; she enjoyed oncology. She said my colon cancer was Stage 2B; but that, for unknown reasons. Stage 3 patients, whose cancers had entered the lymph glands, were surviving better than 2B's like me whose lymph nodes were cancer free.

She echoed the surgeon's opinion: chemotherapy was a good idea because even though tests didn't show residual cancer, there might still be cancer cells in my body. Like the surgeon, she advised me to take six months of "adjuvant" chemotherapy—chemo given to prevent a recurrence of cancer even when tests can't detect any. The agents she suggested—leucovorin, fluorouracil, and oxaliplatin—form a combo called FOLFOX. She said that I didn't have to accept the chemo, but that it would give me a 90% chance to prevent a recurrence of the cancer. The chance without chemo was 70%.

rec. to me by Dr. Lou

I thought my doctors must know better than I what treatment was best for me. I agreed to the chemo. It was scheduled to begin in mid-July. It might be hard on me, the surgeon and oncologist said, but the suffering would be worth it. I talked to my primary care doctor about it, too. He told me he thought I was a strong person, and that very likely chemotherapy wouldn't be difficult for me.

When I was a child, my parents emphasized the importance of being brave, taking on challenges and seeing them through. To get their approval, I almost always did my best to meet the challenge. I think most of us are raised that way.

Shaken by having a body that had failed me, I found myself demoted from adulthood (or maybe I demoted myself). I wanted to be a good child. Unconsciously, I saw my doctors as good adults, good parents. I needed to trust them and I wanted to please them. When they said I needed to suffer chemo to be safe from cancer, I was willing.

Two weeks after surgery, the neat stitches on my surgical wound turned red. The wound was infected—

probably an infection I got during my week in the hospital recovering from surgery. Hospitals are notorious for giving people infections. My surgeon's colleague reopened the wound and cleaned it out—a necessary but very painful treatment that set me screaming. It left a fist-sized hole in my abdomen. (Staring into it was like looking down into a bloody well—really impressive and alarming.)

I couldn't start chemo in July. The toxic chemo drugs would have killed the rapidly dividing healthy cells filling in my wound. It wouldn't be healed until September: I'd have to wait until then to start chemo. Meantime, if I had any cancer cells in my body, the delay would give them time to grow. The oncologist said the delay in starting chemo would reduce my chance of five-year survival of colon cancer from 90% to 55%.

In July and August, I did research on the kind of tumor I had, and on the recommended chemotherapy. Reading the radiologist's report on the tumor, I learned (or relearned—the oncologist had told me already but I'd forgotten) that mine was a "mismatch repair deficient" tumor—an MMRd.[2] I went to the internet to find out more about my "mismatched" tumor. It turns out that in 85% of colon cancer, the immune system "repairs" tumors, eliminating differences in their cells, allowing them to reproduce only identical mutated cells—cells that match. That makes attacking them with a specific chemo agent easier: all the target cells are the same and should respond alike. In contrast, mismatch repair deficient tumors contain many different kinds of mutated cells, which make them much harder to kill. I read that some cancer treatment centers don't advise chemo for mismatch repair deficient tumors.

I brought this up with the oncologist and the surgeon. They acknowledged that some cancer centers advised against chemotherapy after surgery for MMRd's; but they reminded me that besides the two of them, the hospital's tumor board—composed of oncologists, surgeons, radiologists and an oncology nurse—had reviewed my case and also recommended the chemo.

However, my oncologist said, in the light of the mismatched cells, my relative chance for five-year survival was lower than the 55% she'd last estimated. (Five-year "relative survival" is the term used to compare a cancer patient's likelihood of surviving five years to that of cancer-free peers.) The oncologist said that patients who had had homogenous tumors removed and started chemo two months late reduced their relative chance for five-year survival from 90% to 55%. She told me that delaying chemo for a mismatch repair deficient tumor would give me a relative survival percentage of 45-50%—that is, with chemo, I was half as likely to be alive in five years as women my age who were cancer free.

The oncologist told me that the possible side effects of FOLFOX included hair loss, nausea, vomiting, anemia (from new red blood cells being killed off), and neutropenia (fever caused by the chemo killing off new white blood cells); and peripheral neuropathy (numb or burning hands and feet). Afterward, the friend with me remembered her mentioning all these effects, but I didn't.

When I looked up possible side effects of FOLFOX on line, most of the information sounded entirely new to me.[3]

Patients treated with FOLFOX have a 70% chance of suffering peripheral neuropathy. Of that 70%, half suffered the hand and foot pain for several years after chemo concluded. I mentioned this to a friend who is a primary care doctor. Some of his patients had had post-chemo neuropathy. "The pain in their feet is excruciating," he said.

I considered my feet—very useful. Handy for walking. I considered my hands. As a writer, I'd typed all my manuscripts for so many years that it seemed my ideas were stored in my hands and poured out of my fingertips. I wasn't sure I could adapt to another way or working, especially if I were also nauseous, anemic, vomiting, losing my hair in clumps, and feverish from a lack of white blood cells.

On the other hand, a friend told me of a sixty-year-old man she knew, a dentist, who'd done the FOLFOX chemo with no difficulty and kept working full time throughout. He hadn't had peripheral neuropathy, and had had no recurrence of cancer in eight years. To be fair, I had to admit I might come through chemo like him. But maybe not.

I saw the "nurse navigator" at the hospital. Her job was to help patients find other services there—a yoga class, the dietician's office, a survivors' meeting group. It seemed to me, though, that her real role was to scare people into chemo. She implied that I'd die if I didn't do it. I broke down and wept in the hospital corridor. She smiled. I think she was trying to look compassionate and in command of my future. The cancer hadn't brought me to tears, but the thought of the chemo did. In the months before the colon cancer diagnosis and surgery, anemia had been the worst of the suffering. As I lay in bed, all the emotional tones and colors that flowed through my life blanched to an infinitely slow procession of identical instants. The prospect of getting anemia from the chemo overwhelmed me.

I e-mailed the surgeon, arguing that, since chemotherapy lowers immune function, using it to cure cancer isn't logical. He replied that according to statistics, it would improve my chances to survive. We batted our conflicting views back and forth over the internet. Finally, I told him that statistics weren't the issue. Right or wrong, after having been terribly ill and now feeling good, I couldn't bear the idea of deliberately making myself sick all over again with FOLFOX. He responded with great sympathy and stopped pushing me to do chemo.

I was still weak. I concentrated on building up my stamina, taking longer and longer walks. When I walked too far I'd get severe cramps and be afraid of collapsing. The wound had to be checked and cleaned at the hospital three times a week for several months. A small but very expensive pump called a Vac suctioned fluids out of it 24 hours a day. I wore the pump like a shoulder bag during the day, hoping all the normal people on the street wouldn't notice the tubing and realize I wasn't like them, that there was something wrong with me. At night I kept the Vac on the floor next to my bedside table. When its battery got low and it needed to be plugged into an outlet, it would beep at me. Every two days the wound care nurses, tremendous morale builders, marveled at my progress. They were encouraging about chemo. They all thought I'd handle it well—except for one rebel who said, "Chemotherapy! You'll love it! It's so good! Hah-hah! I'd better say no more. Maybe the walls have ears."

I kept getting stronger. Pain from healing was strangely different from the pain of cancer. During the cancer I'd felt an insidious sour emptiness, as if in every breath, grayness, disgust, and distaste for life was slowly growing, covering up all of me. In healing, there was pain, too, but every twinge felt cleansing and hopeful.

On the internet, I read about a Hungarian doctor who in the 1950s claimed to cure cancer patients with a diet that included five pounds of beets a day. To prevent a return of cancer, every morning I ate a tablespoon of evaporated beet juice powder mixed in yogurt. The vendor claimed that the daily tablespoon was the nutritional equivalent of eating five pounds of fresh beets.

On November 9, 2012, my wound fully healed, feeling great, trusting in the power of beets, I had my six-month follow-up. I got devastating news. The CT scan showed that two tumors, new lymph nodes a quarter inch in diameter by an inch and a half long, had formed between my lungs. The oncologist said that radiation would be useless against them, and that chemotherapy couldn't cure them. She recommended a six months chemo course anyway—"palliative chemotherapy"—the name oncologists give to chemotherapy that can't cure. She said using it would extend my life by twenty months. The chemo combination would be FOLFOX, the exact same chemo I'd rejected in July.

The oncologist said that to confirm the diagnosis, she could do a biopsy—but that it would hurt. I turned it down—I'd read that biopsies can cause tumors to spread. She arranged for me to have a PET scan and a follow-up appointment with her for November 27.

The clear cold certainty of the numbers I'd clung to in my cancer journey—first my 90% chance of five-year survival, than my 55% chance, then my 45-50% chance— had melted like an ice cube in my hands—melted down to zero.

Two: A Letter and a Phone Call

Four years earlier my husband, who had smoked heavily between the ages of 14 and 60, had been diagnosed with inoperable cancer in one lung and damage from smoking in the other. He no longer smoked. He was eighty years old, but strong and active. People usually thought he was in his late sixties. His doctors had recommended chemotherapy and radiation: one thought he'd have a 30% chance to beat the cancer. But he had kidney damage that the chemo would probably make worse. He knew if he survived the cancer, there was a risk that his kidneys would fail and he'd end up on dialysis. He left a note for his kidney doctor letting her know he had cancer and asking what her experience had been with her patients who took chemo. More than a week later, after several more requests for her response, she phoned him to say she couldn't generalize and had no advice. Bill knew two friends with bad kidneys who had told him that getting the dialysis treatments three days a week and recovering from them four days a week had made their life not worth living.

Bill said he didn't want to ever be a burden to anyone. I said he'd never be a burden. He said, "I don't want to live being pushed to dialysis with an oxygen tank on my wheel chair." He refused chemo and radiation. I searched on the internet and found twenty or so potential natural cures, bought them, and urged him to take them. He looked at the mound of capsules by his plate and protested, "How am I going to have room to eat anything?" I think if I'd focused on his diet, not on capsules, he would have been better off.

All the expensive capsules failed Bill. Now that I had cancer, I knew better than to waste time on them. But as I read about new curative regimens, most seemed dubious, or so complicated and demanding—as well as unproven—that I wasn't willing to try them either.

I don't remember why, but after a few days of research, I Googled "cancer" and "five pounds of carrots." A memo opened up as a page of a family website. In the memo, a man named Ralph Cole said that he had cured ten small squamous cell tumors on his chest in eight weeks. He'd done this back in 2006, by juicing five pounds of carrots daily and drinking the resulting five cups of juice. (One pound equals .45 kilos and one U.S. cup is .24 liters.)

Months earlier, in 2005, two larger tumors had protruded outward from his neck. They resembled hard-boiled eggs in shape and firmness. Biopsies at a hospital indicated they were both cancerous. He allowed the physicians to schedule surgery for him, which was to take place four months later. At the same time, he began juicing carrots at the advice of an acquaintance. He juiced three pounds of carrots a day. The tumors didn't grow, but they didn't disappear. Because they hadn't grown, he was able to persuade the medical staff to skip the surgery. But because they hadn't gone away and also because he was the father of young children and wanted to make sure he would be around for them, he consented to radiation treatments and chemotherapy.

During and after the six weeks of conventional treatments, he continued juicing carrots. The two big tumors finally disappeared several months after radiation and chemotherapy concluded. Something in the combination of radiation, chemotherapy, and three cups per day of carrot juice got rid of the tumors temporarily. But the radiation treatments also caused him to lose his teeth and permanently damaged his ability to salivate and swallow. When he lost his ability to swallow, he had wanted to stop the radiation treatments, but his doctors insisted that if he stopped, he would jeopardize his recovery and invalidate a study they had placed him in. They also wrongly insisted that his ability to swallow would completely return within about a week of the end of the radiation treatments. He was hospitalized for a while, unable to eat or drink without a tube through his nose to his stomach. And the cure didn't last, either. Four months after the tumors on his neck disappeared, ten new ones emerged on his chest.

He could see and feel them under his skin. Each was small, about the size of a grain of rice. He returned to drinking three eight ounce glasses of fresh carrot juice daily—the juice from three pounds of carrots. Once again, the tumors didn't grow, but they didn't shrink either. He showed them to a nurse he knew and asked her what she thought he should do. She said he should go back to the hospital and receive more treatments. Given what he had been through, this did not sound good to him.

Instead, he upped his juicing from three pounds of carrots per day, which had given him three cups of juice, to five pounds, which produced five cups of juice. The tumors appeared to shrink the first day, and even more the second. And they *had* shrunk. All but one disappeared within six weeks. The largest was gone in eight weeks. To be sure all the cancer cells were really gone, for another month he continued juicing five pounds of carrots daily. Then he gave up juicing. This time, no new tumors appeared.

His memo suggested that, although the experience of just one person gave no guarantee of success, it might be worthwhile for other cancer sufferers to try carrots.

The objective tone of his memo impressed me. He didn't promise that carrots could cure all cancers. He wasn't selling carrots, juicers, vacuum-sealing carrot containers, or amazing miracle carrot seed. He wasn't selling anything.

The memo contained his phone number. I called. He told me he'd used just ordinary carrots from the supermarket to make his juice. In the seven years since his carrot cure, the cancer hadn't returned. He hadn't ever gone back to juicing. He believed five pounds of carrots daily were the threshold for eliminating cancer: more might be good, but for certain, less wouldn't do for a normal size and weight adult. He had advised a few people in his church with a variety of cancers to try the carrot juicing, and said that several were seeing improvement in their symptoms. He sounded honest.

I bought a juicer the next day—on November 16, 2012—and started drinking carrot juice, five cups daily.

Three: The Shooter Misses

The two tumors were between my lungs, not inside them. So far, they didn't interfere with my breathing. Except for short stabbing attacks of grief, I was feeling great. I could walk without my strength giving way and cramps starting in my abdomen. I could ride my bike eight miles once again. Without treatment, I probably still had some months of continued good health ahead of me. Should I sacrifice those good months for the uncertain promise of a longer life?

As before, I still couldn't believe in making myself sick to make myself well. I couldn't believe in destroying my immune system to defeat cancer. At moments I felt I heard an inner voice warning me that if I even started on the road to chemotherapy, it would be the end for me. The voice was matter-of-fact and very convincing. I listened to it.

My friends and family accepted my decision against

chemo, but it alarmed most of them. They couldn't believe that conventional treatments wouldn't be beneficial. After all, if they weren't, why did they exist and why did all oncologists prescribe them?

My sister flew across the country from Connecticut to go to the November 27 appointment with me. I was quite sure bad news was in store. When we got to the clinic, the oncologist was running two hours behind schedule. The receptionist knew about the delay, but didn't tell us—not because she was a bad person, but because the routines of the clinic had never been set up with consideration for patients' feelings. As the minutes dragged, my mood went from apprehension to anxiety to rage. We could have asked when we arrived if the oncologist would be on time. If we'd been told the length of the delay, we could have left a cell phone number with the receptionist and gone out for a walk or a coffee to relieve tension. (We finally did that after waiting an hour and a half.)

We saw the oncologist. She apologized for her lateness. I suggested that informing patients of known delays should be made a policy in the clinic. She agreed and had me speak to the clinic manager, who promised improvements. Then we got on to the gloomy business of the day. The PET scan had confirmed the earlier CT. Two tumors, the same size as they'd been in the CT, and some "spots." The PET scan showed the spots and the tumors were growing rapidly and quickly taking up the radioactive sugar. Colon cancer usually grows slowly; the oncologist believed the metastasis to the lungs had occurred before surgery, but had been undetectable then. She retroactively revised her original staging of the colon tumor. In June, I probably hadn't had Stage 2B colon cancer; I'd probably already had Stage 4.

The palliative chemo she was recommending could lengthen my life by twenty months. If I didn't accept FOLFOX, my first symptoms—fatigue, breathlessness, a cough—would probably begin within seven months to a year. I said I still didn't want chemo. My sister, alarmed to see me burning my bridges, asked the oncologist how much I'd reduce the benefit of the chemo if I put it off six weeks, until after the next CT. The oncologist said the delay wouldn't make much difference. I liked her a lot for that, and also for having told me straight out that chemo couldn't cure my cancer. My sister's question—how much would I reduce the benefit of conventional treatment through postponing it?—is a valuable one for anyone who wants to try a natural cure or ponder a proposed treatment before accepting it.

Apparently carrots weren't working, but I kept on juicing them every day. I didn't look for any other cure. I think maybe we have a "backup brain"—one we use for emergencies when the nimble, calculating, doubting, discontented rational brain finds no solutions. My backup brain told me to juice carrots, so I went on drinking the juice, without much hope, but also without question.

In December, I consulted the surgeon. He recommended chemotherapy. I asked him how long he thought I had to live. Two to three years, he said.

Ralph Cole phoned me to see how I was doing. I was

very moved by his kindness to a total stranger. I told him about the rapid growth of the tumors and that the carrot juice cure apparently wasn't working. "The oncologist said PET shows the tumors are growing rapidly," he pointed out, "and yet she also said they aren't any bigger than they were three weeks earlier. Maybe they grew in the week before you started carrots, but since then they've been shrinking." It did seem contradictory that the tumors were growing rapidly but no bigger than they had been three weeks earlier. Another of life's mysteries.

I got through the Christmas and New Year's holidays with friends politely not mentioning my disease—the invisible elephant in the room, towering over the Christmas tree. Since no one saw it but me, I could almost pretend it wasn't there.

On January 9, the oncologist shared my next CT results with me. Surprised and cautiously pleased, she gave me good news. The two tumors hadn't grown; in fact, they'd shrunk slightly. She didn't recommend chemotherapy. I didn't need to stay in Portland. I could do what I wanted—fly to Guatemala for the winter. I got to Guatemala where the carrots are gigantic and very sweet. I kept on juicing carrots. I thought that maybe, they were curing me.

In March 2013 in Guatemala City, I had a new CT scan. I brought the Guatemalan oncologist the X-ray and the report from the lab in a big white envelope. I was dying to see them—those were my results, after all, which I had paid for—but I didn't, because of a lifetime of conditioning in respect—the results were for the doctor, not for me, the humble body in question. I sat across from him in his office, my eyes fixed on the envelope, which he didn't open for what seemed an eternity. Meantime he asked me once again, as he'd done on my first visit with him, if there were any circumstances *at all* in which I'd agree to chemotherapy. I told him I couldn't think of any.

"At the bottom of my heart," he said, "I know that if I got cancer I would refuse chemotherapy. I've seen too many awful effects from it."

At last he opened the envelope. The new CT scan showed no swollen lymph nodes—the previously enlarged cancerous ones had shrunk further. They were normal. I think this means that I no longer had cancer—but he didn't tell me that, so I went on juicing carrots daily.

In mid-July 2013, I returned to Portland. I had a CT on July 30. On August 1, I got the results from my original oncologist: "Little change from January" and: "No Sign of Cancer."

Six weeks after diagnosis, two very aggressive tumors between the lungs had stopped growing. In three more months, all pulmonary lymph nodes were normal. In another three and a half months, the same result worded differently: no sign of cancer.

Being diagnosed with cancer that was expected to kill me, and then being entirely free from it was an extraordinary experience—joyous! As Winston Churchill once noted, "There is nothing more exhilarating than to be shot at with no result."

For the first time, I told my oncologist that I'd been using carrots as my weapon against cancer. I explained that I hadn't told her earlier because I figured she'd be skeptical.

She smiled and said she'd always thought I was the kind of person who'd try some natural alternative against the cancer. "And I'm not skeptical. I believe there are many natural substances that can attack cancer. I can't recommend any in particular, though, because we don't have statistics on their success."

I was feeling too good that day to ask the obvious question—why aren't statistics kept on those who cure themselves of cancer without chemotherapy and radiation?

Every year the big drug companies spend nearly twice as much on advertising as they do on research—including more than $61,000 per individual U.S. doctor.[1] Besides that, almost all cancer research spending focuses on the problems chemotherapy and radiation cause, or on minor differences between drugs already in use.

Compared with those R and D and marketing billions, how much could it cost to follow up all patients, to know what their outcomes are? A substantial number of those who reject chemotherapy and radiation may have tried alternative cures and died of their cancer. Others may have tried something that worked—as I did. Wouldn't it be worthwhile to know what both these groups have tried, and to use this information to guide investigations into natural treatments? Why isn't it done?

I asked that question of an old friend, an inventor of

medical devices. He said, "Who is going to pay for it? Drug companies can't make money selling carrots."

Four: Falcarinol and Luteolin

It turns out that there is strong scientific evidence for carrots as an anti-cancer treatment. Carrots contain an amazing number of compounds, and not all their effects and interactions are known.[1] Two, falcarinol and luteolin, have been studied for over ten years. Both have strong anti-cancer effects.

Falcarinol is a compound in all carrots which prevents fungi from attacking their roots. It's also present in celery, parsnips, parsley, fennel, and ginseng.

For years, Dr. Kirsten Brandt, at the University of Newcastle-on-Tyne in the U.K., has investigated carrots and falcarinol. In many experiments, lab rats and mice were injected with carcinogens. Dr. Brandt found that, compared to mice or rats eating their normal chow, those supplemented with carrots or falcarinol developed a third fewer large tumors.[2] (This is important: small tumors don't kill; it's those that grow larger that are the killers.)

In Dr. Brandt's lab, the experimental animals ate blanched, shredded, freeze-dried carrots equal to 20% of the calories in their diets.

The human equivalent of the dose her lab animals ate is slightly over pound and a half of carrots daily. Five pounds of carrots, the amount Ralph Cole and I used, is three times that. Dr. Brandt has not done any experiments on people, and of course, human biology and rats' aren't necessarily the same. However, if what is true for rats is also true for humans, people consuming a pound and a half of carrots daily could reduce large tumor formation by a third. And it would be reasonable to suppose that three times that amount might eliminate tumors entirely.

Falcarinol is present in carrots in tiny quantities—a liter of juice from orange carrots contains only 13 milligrams.[3] (To get an idea of how small an amount this is, visualize a gram, which is only about a US quarter teaspoon measure. A milligram is only a thousandth of that!) Five cups of carrot juice have around 17-mg. falcarinol.

Another anti-cancer compound in carrots, much more studied than falcarinol, is luteolin. Luteolin has amazing benefits for health.[4] In 2008, the journal *Molecules* summed up its anti-cancer effects: "Luteolin displays specific anti-inflammatory and anticarcinogenic effects, which can only partly be explained by its antioxidant and free radical scavenging capacities. Luteolin can delay or block the development of cancer cells in vitro and in vivo by protection from carcinogenic stimuli, by inhibition of tumor cell proliferation, by induction of cell cycle arrest and by induction of apoptosis via intrinsic and extrinsic signaling pathways. When compared to other flavonoids, luteolin was usually among the most effective..."

Besides its presence in carrots, luteolin is also found in parsley, wheatgrass, lemongrass, green peppers, celery, chamomile, yarrow, rooibos tea, thyme, peppermint, basil, artichokes, citrus fruits, and green onion leaves.[5] In a usual diet, Americans consume a milligram of luteolin daily—a tiny amount. There are 75-mg. luteolin in five pounds of carrots—75 times the usual American consumption. It's possible to buy purified luteolin in 100 mg. capsules, but luteolin is much better absorbed when it's taken with its companion nutrients in a whole food. According to the *Journal of Nutrition*, "No single antioxidant can replace the combination of natural phytochemicals in fruits and vegetables to achieve their health benefits. The evidence suggests that antioxidants or bioactive compounds are best acquired through whole-food consumption, not from expensive dietary supplements."[6]

Five: Juicing Carrots

Here's how to do it.

Buy or borrow a juicer. You can find them used on ebay. Any kind will work, but a blender won't. (If you disregard this point and use a blender, you'll end up with a lot of mashed carrot, no juice, and a broken blender.)

Check reviews on the internet before you buy a juicer, and get a sturdy machine: the cheapest break down under heavy use. Some reviews claim that certain types of juicers make juice too fast, heating the juice and oxidizing it. I believe that with any type of juicer the resulting juice is plenty good enough to cure cancer.

Every day it took me about fifteen minutes to juice the carrots, begin to drink the juice, and clean the juicer. I used ordinary carrots, not organic ones. Any color carrots will work. The important thing for the cure is that the carrots are fresh. You can be sure you're getting fresh ones if you buy them with their green tops. Break off the greens right away. If you don't, they'll draw nutrients and water out of the carrot roots, making them less nutritive. Scrub the carrots very lightly to get them clean. Don't peel them—you'll lose half or more of the anti-cancer ingredient falcarinol, which is highest in the carrot skin. Cut off any bad spots. There are different levels of falcarinol in different varieties of carrots. Purple carrots, if you can find them, have six times the amount of the falcarinol in orange carrots, but the orange ones work fine. Maybe for someone very ill, who can't drink five cups of juice daily, it would be worth it to search out purple carrots.

Don't buy carrots that look brown around the stem; they aren't freshly picked. Also avoid buying carrots that have a greenish area at the stem end; the green part is bitter. It appears on carrots that have been planted too high, so that when they're growing, they get sunburned. If you do buy carrots with a greenish top, just chop the green part off and discard it.

Cut the carrots into pieces that will fit your juicer. They will make about five cups of juice (1.2 liters). They'll also make a lot of pulp. If the pulp is quite moist, you can run it through a juicer twice to extract more juice. The pulp is a good addition to dog food or in compost if you have a garden. There's some falcarinol in the pulp, but you will get plenty of it in the juice and don't need to eat the pulp. Cleaning the juicer parts only requires scrubbing them lightly and rinsing them off in cold water for a matter of seconds.

Ralph took his carrot juice straight and didn't mix

anything with it. He drank it all as soon as he made it. Many people don't report this, but I found the carrots had a very strong laxative effect if I drank all the juice at once, so I drank mine throughout the day, usually on an empty stomach, when absorption is better.

Keep the juice in the refrigerator in glass jars with lids. If you are pressed for time in the morning, you can prepare the carrots at night. Wash and cut them into pieces that fit into the juicer, then put them back into the refrigerator in a plastic bag. In the morning, you'll be able to make the juice in about ten minutes. If you take the juice with you to work, use a thermos or keep it covered in a dark place. Make sure to drink all the juice in one day.

I usually spiced up the juice with an apple and fresh ginger, and sometimes parsley leaves, a celery stalk, melon or other fruit. Ralph used only carrots to make his juice.

Ralph found that three cups of plain carrot juice daily stopped his cancer from growing, but they didn't eliminate it. If you can't manage to drink five cups daily, just three cups will probably arrest the growth of tumors. If you are very ill and unable to eat, even a cup of juice may improve your health and make it possible for you to gradually increase the amount you can drink. Assuming you have no trouble drinking, whatever you add to your juice, the essential thing is to always use five pounds of carrots. Small people may get by with less juice. Those weighing over 160 pounds (70 kg.) should drink several more cups daily.

High heat destroys falcarinol and its companion compound falcarindiol. Drinking bottled pasteurized juice from a store will give you the benefit of luteolin, which isn't heat sensitive, but not the benefit of carrot enzymes or falcarinol and its related compounds. There are additional compounds in carrots that have yet to be explored medically and that are probably available only in raw juice.

Ralph Cole skipped juicing one day a week—but never more. In eight months I skipped five days in a row three times, because I was traveling and didn't have access to a juicer. It won't hurt to miss a few times, but making juice your top priority nearly every day is essential to a cure. Focus and commitment is a vital part of winning against cancer.

Half an hour after you drink the juice, falcarinol can be found in your bloodstream. Its concentration reaches a peak in the blood two hours after drinking.[1] If you are sick from chemo or radiation and it's difficult to drink, have as much as you can manage, on an empty stomach for better absorption.

Beta-carotene in carrots can change your skin tone and turn it lightly orange. I thought my skin looked better that way—tanned—rather than with its usual Portland pallor. The orange color is a harmless effect that will go away when you stop juicing. If you have diabetes and are concerned about sugar, you might substitute celery for part of the carrot juice. Celery sometimes has double or triple the amount of falcarinol in carrots, but sometimes much less. It also has apigenin, which has been discovered to have its own very strong anti-cancer effects. Beta-carotene is not Vitamin A; it's a precursor to

Vitamin A. That is, the body converts what beta-carotene it needs to Vitamin A and eliminates the rest. There is little danger of a Vitamin A overdose or a strain on the liver from eating carrots.[2]

Besides hearing from people who will urgently tell you carrots are bad for your liver, you are no doubt going to hear from those who are sure you are getting "too much" sugar from carrots and "feeding the cancer." The benefits of the anti-cancer ingredients in carrots more than offset any problem from sugar. True, it's important to avoid refined sugar and empty calories from sweets; but carrots, and most fruits, are rich in flavonoids and polyphenols that more than make up from any excess of sugar.

All your cells live on glucose. Cancerous cells are more efficient than healthy cells at taking the sugar from the bloodstream. To deprive cancer cells of glucose, you'd have to deprive all your normal cells of sugar first, and they (and you) would die. As the sugar from the carrot juice enters cancer cells, the falcarinol, luteolin and other ingredients that wake up the immune system enter, too. People who warn you to avoid carrots because they have too much sugar are like someone telling you "Don't put that piece of cheese in the mousetrap! You're going to feed the mice!"

I recommend using only carrot juice from one scan to the next, so if there is a decrease in tumor growth rate or size you will know what caused it. I think the right time for a scan is after six to eight weeks of carrot juicing. Ralph thinks a scan will detect improvement in four weeks. Ralph cautions that even if carrot juice isn't shrinking your tumor, it is probably keeping it from growing as fast as it otherwise would, and that before you give up on carrot juice you should increase the regularity with which you juice and the total amount you drink. I believe that if in eight weeks your scan results don't improve, you should take another approach to your treatment besides carrots.

If you attempt the carrot cure, you will be using carrots medicinally—consuming much more of them than anyone would normally. In addition to carrot juice, you should have a healthy diet—little meat or processed foods and lots of fruits and vegetables. However, I recommend making carrots the only dietary ingredient you take medicinally. It's possible that simultaneously forcing down every exotic natural anti-cancer treatment you've ever heard of might speed your cure. However, not all of them are well researched and you can wind up spending a lot of money very fast on things you know nothing about, increasing your stress, panic and doubt.

Carrots alone cured me. There are many cellular pathways that contribute to curing cancer—but some of them may be incompatible. In using the "everything but the kitchen sink" approach you might cause traffic congestion, with one anti-cancer treatment blocking or canceling the effects of another. Another possible problem is that consuming many such ingredients, you may develop a sensitivity to one. Your whole body itches, and you know you have to give something up—but which ingredient is the one to avoid? You have no idea. (One woman with such an itch had used a number of anti-cancer ingredients for months, and had just started carrot juicing. She thought carrot juice consumption had caused the itch. I told her she was the first person to mention any problem with carrots. She quit garlic, which she had been eating for a long time in large quantities, and the itch went away.)

Another possible problem: You take an anti-cancer smorgasbord for six weeks, learn you haven't stopped the cancer, and fall into panic and despair. Maybe one of the ingredients you used would have been effective, except that you weren't getting enough of it—but you have no idea which. And then, having already "tried everything," you have no idea what's failing, what's succeeding, or what do next.

Botanists and research biochemists may know what treatments are synergistic and which incompatible. I don't. I suppose other foods or spices containing luteolin and falcarinol will be compatible with carrots. All I'm sure about is that using carrots, and no other foods as medicine, worked for me. I juiced five pounds of carrots almost daily for eight months, and now I have no detectable cancer. It was simple. It was safe. For me and some others, it worked.

If you try another natural remedy, investigate it thoroughly through online research and try to find studies from respected universities that validate the approach. Use formal and specific scientific names to get the best results, and look up your kind of cancer by name. For instance, when I looked up cancer and carrots together, I found almost no information; but in an online search for "luteolin" together with "prostate cancer", I found many interesting studies. Looking up simply "natural cancer cures," I came across one very dismal litany than ran something like this: "There is no proof that mushrooms can cure cancer: there is no proof that broccoli can cure cancer; there is no evidence that curcumin can cure cancer." For the anonymous writer of the article "proof" obviously could come only from double-blinded clinical trials which will never be undertaken. But if you search for specific cancers with vegetables, fruits or spices, you will find plenty of evidence for their anti-cancer effects.

While I juiced the carrots I ate my normal diet, which included thin pancakes stuffed with fruit; pasta; pizza (thin crust pizza with minimal cheese and lots of vegetables); yogurt, cheese, a little milk, very occasional red meat; chicken, eggs, salad, black beans with onion, garlic and cilantro; tortillas, and a small piece of chocolate most days. The first seven weeks I was using carrots, almost every day I had a Trader Joe's mini ice cream cone (or two!). I drank two or three glasses of red wine a week. I never had sodas, chips, or any other junk food. I took a B complex vitamin, two probiotics daily and occasionally extra Vitamin B12 sublingually. I didn't take vitamins A, C, D, or E. High D levels are supposed to help prevent cancer, but Guatemala is very sunny, so I believed I didn't need any additional D from capsules. In some cases Vitamin E as alpha-tocopherol stimulates cancer.[3] I didn't take folic acid.[4] Folates from greens are healthy, but folic acid, which is a synthetic folate, can be cancerous.

Anti-cancer compounds in isolation, in too low or too high amounts, (for instance the use of luteolin tablets against endometrial cancer) can have consequences entirely opposite from what we hope for. The most prudent course is to get nutrients from food.

Since inflammation in the body stimulates cancer, it would be a good idea to eliminate inflammatory foods from your diet and add those that are anti-inflammatory.

All the time I was juicing, people who didn't know I had cancer commented on how healthy I looked. My skin started looking radiant. Acne went away. I got strong fingernails for the first time in my life. My hair grew better. I didn't get any colds at all: I was used to having several a year that could hang on for weeks and make me miserable. Muscle aches vanished. Despite being aware that I might die from cancer, I felt unusually happy most of the time. I think I was learning to ignore things that don't matter and to appreciate the most basic things in life—the feeling of a breeze on my skin; the stars in the sky; and love.

For Ralph Cole, carrots were effective medicine. He has been cancer free for over seven years since his carrot juice dosing months, and he's only rarely juiced carrots since. I hope that like him, I'm not only "free of signs of cancer," but have put the disease behind me.

As a follow-up to my July 2013 CT scan, I had a colonoscopy and an endoscopy in early September 2013. They showed no cancer and no inflammation in my intestine. Before the procedures, though, the gastroenterologist pressed me toward more cancer treatment. "Now why don't you have chemotherapy, just in case you have a little cancer to mop up?"

I told him I'd already mopped it up—with carrots.

Six: Treating the Community of Cells

Therapeia is the ancient Greek word for healing. What we call chemotherapy—treating cancer by injecting people with chemicals never naturally found in the human body—is more a chemical assault than a therapy. It began as a wartime experiment in the 1940s. Researchers with the United States military noticed reports that battlefield exposure in World War I to a chemical weapon, mustard gas, had stopped the growth of soldiers' rapidly dividing white blood cells. It occurred to them that mustard gas might also work against rapidly growing cancerous cells. Breathing in mustard gas irritated the lungs, but as a liquid, it could be infused into a vein. The immediate effect on tumors was dramatic. They shrank rapidly and even disappeared completely. Unfortunately, success from this approach was temporary for almost all types of cancer. Soon new tumors, or undetectable remains of the old ones, grew again. In spite of its tremendously high rate of failure, in over sixty years, the strategy of using toxic chemicals to destroy tumors has remained the basic medical approach to cancer.

People often believe that the expensive and difficult is better than the cheap and easy. It seems laughable to suggest that the humble carrot can do more for you than radiation or chemo. However, in the world of cancer treatment, the low-cost and gentle can be better and more effective than the most expensive and highly recommended new drugs. We don't understand that because we don't think much about the nature of our own bodies.

A carrot is not only a low-priced, mildly sweet crunchy orange treat fortunately well shaped for enclosure in a plastic bag. A carrot is an organism that has grown and evolved over thousands of years, changing to meet changing environments, developing chemicals to defeat many enemies attacking them from underground and from the air. Over many millennia, too, our bodies and our diets have adapted, using these same chemicals to defend us against our attackers. In a sense you could say our bodies have learned from carrots. Carrots are smart! They've had thousands of years to work on their chemistry, and haven't made a misstep and gone extinct. Admittedly they have no diplomas, small vocabularies, and no brain—but they possess innate intelligence, and that allows them to doctor us.

Just as we rarely stop to think of a carrot as a living thing, in the stillness of a mirror's view we never see our own bodies' internal never-ceasing dynamism. That makes it easy to conceive of a tumor as being like a large rock that's fallen through the roof into our house and needs to be dynamited. Bomb the rock, and when the dust settles, we'll rebuild. That's the approach of chemo and radiation—for half a century our favorite weapons in "the war against cancer." Unfortunately our house, the body, is vulnerable: the dust is alive and full of seeds. If it flies instead of settling, the damage to the house can be fatal.

It's interesting that in their different ways both chemotherapy and radiation have had a long history tied to weapons of war. More than half a century has gone by while we pay over and over again to win the fight against cancer—with never a solid victory in sight.

When I found that colon cancer had metastasized to my lungs, I determined not to think of it as a dreaded omnipotent enemy that had control of my body. Scientifically, as well as psychologically, I was right.

Naturally when we learn we have a tumor, we want it gone immediately, and sometimes what doctors call the "tumor burden"—its size—must be reduced by standard treatments before it overwhelms us: the advance of cancer doesn't always leave natural treatments sufficient time to do their work. But the tumor is not the root of cancer,—it's only a symptom. Cancer is a systemic failure, a breakdown of the body's regulation of cell growth and cell destruction.[1] Nutritional research shows that dietary ingredients alone can restore the body's power to regulate cell creation and death.

Until the early 1990s, the focus of cancer research

was on tumors and individual cancer cells. Then researchers realized that without the cooperation of normal, healthy cells, cancerous ones couldn't grow. The neighbors of cancer cells permit or deny their growth. What controls the neighborhood are cellular switches that regulate the expression of genes. Some of our genes are "onco-genes"—genes that naturally promote cancer. Others are naturally cancer suppressors.

Imagine a young delinquent living in your neighborhood. What he can get away with depends on the reactions of his noncriminal neighbors. They notice his activities and phone each other about him. After a while, some of them may prefer to quit worrying about the guy, turn off the phone, settle back on the couch and watch TV. Others may be crime-tolerant enablers. One or two may be converted by his talk and join him in a life of crime. Others may report him to the police. Still others may organize the whole neighborhood to disarm him and get him locked up.

Similarly in the body, a delinquent cell—a cancerous one—lives in a neighborhood. What it can get away with depends on the cross talk—the signaling—among its noncriminal neighbors. Chemicals carried in the blood can change cell signaling and the expression of genes.[2] In each cell, the genes are wound like thread around protein spools called histones. Temporary but often long-lasting settings on the histones control gene expression. Chemicals, including nutrients, affect the spools and can switch on or put to sleep cells' awareness of what's going on around them and what ought to be done about it.

The study of the cell signaling that controls expression of genes is called epigenetics. The prefix "epi" comes from the Greek for "on top of." Epigenetics rules genes. Like our genes, the settings for our epigenetic switches are inherited from our parents. Our genes only change in the rare case of a mutation, but epigenetic switching is reversible. That's why twins who are identical at birth may be very different in appearance, personality, and health by the time they reach adulthood.[3]

An epigenetic switch may be set to turn on the activity of an oncogene—a gene that promotes the formation of cancer. It may be reset to turn the oncogene off. A switch may be set to stimulate cell division, or to tell cells to die. In the body's ceaseless conversation with itself, the chances for change end only with death. A single health-building food can adjust the conversation in hundreds of ways, while a manufactured synthetic drug may work only one way—not enough to change things.

In 2012, in the journal *Nutrition and Cancer*, cancer researchers considering the dynamism of the body, wrote:

> Four decades after U.S. President Nixon officially declared the "War on Cancer," the overall rates of cancer have not substantially changed. ...Why are we losing the war against cancer? ...We argue that the primary cause is too narrow a focus in the effort to develop a cancer drug for a single target... Extensive research within the past half-century has revealed that cancer is caused by a dysregulation of as many as 500 different gene products. Most natural products target multiple gene products and thus are ideally

suited for prevention and treatment of many chronic diseases, including cancer.[4]

Researchers in nutritional epigenetics have found that some fruits, vegetables, herbs and spices can wake up the cells of the immune system and cause them to kill cancer.

You could compare beneficial nutri-epigenetic effects on the body's genes to the work of a piano tuner. It's the same piano before and after the tune-up, but beforehand, with some notes set way high and others silenced, the piano doesn't work right, and the music goes awry.

Carrots are one of the foods that, used in large enough quantities, as medicine, can achieve this re-tuning. They might do it for you. If they don't, other foods may. Avocados, cabbage, broccoli sprouts, spinach, grapes, apple peel, lemons, strawberries, black raspberries, turmeric, rosemary, cinnamon and many others have anti-cancer effects.[5]

The difficulty is in the details—learning how much it takes of any of them, or a particular combination of them, to cure cancer. The advantage of using carrots as medicine is that in a number of people, the same quantity of carrot juice—five cups—has cured cancer quickly and in a similar time frame. (More carrot juice daily wouldn't hurt, and of course it's possible that some people with cancer might need even more.)

You'll remember that when Dr. Kirsten Brandt fed her mice and rats carrots or falcarinol, they developed fewer large tumors. Tumors grow large only when they are able to stimulate new blood vessels to form and bring them nutrients. That process is called angiogenesis—"angio" from the Greek word meaning container or vessel, and "genesis" from the Greek word for development.

One of the ways carrots reduce cancer is through "anti-angiogenesis." Dr. William Li of Harvard Medical School, has done much research on anti-angiogenic foods—foods that stop tumors from forming their network of new blood vessels. In a TED talk "Can We Eat to Starve Cancer?" Dr. Li describes his laboratory's study of anti-angiogenic foods.[6] Anti-angiogenic foods change our epigenetic signaling and thereby save our lives. Carrots are one of the best of these foods.

We know we can't change our genes. That can make us fatalistic about our life expectancy and unaware of the importance of our individual choices. But nutri-epigenetics is as important in our lives as our genetics.

Speaking at a leadership conference in 2008, Craig Venter, the first scientist to sequence the human genome, de-emphasized the importance of genetics. "Human biology is much more complicated than we imagine," he said. "Everybody talks about the genes they got from their mother and father, for this trait or the other. But in reality, those genes have very little impact on life outcomes. Our biology is way too complicated for that and deals with hundreds of thousands of independent factors. Genes are absolutely not our fate."[7]

Tumors begin from mutated genes in single cells, but

it's signaling problems in the body that permit the growth of those single cells. They form tumors when normal cells lose their capacity to recognize them, or the defective cells lose their ability to respond to signals.[8] Though the immune system is still present, it has become part of the problem rather than the solution. Dietary changes can restore its normal functioning.[9]

In his essay "Why Cancer and Inflammation?" Dr. Seth Rakoff-Nahoum, Professor of Immunobiology at Yale University School of Medicine, discusses the causes of cancer. He says most cancers derive from irritants that cause long-term inflammation. The irritation might come from a viral or bacterial infection, smoking, particular foods, or exposure to pollutants. The body's innate response is to send immune system cells to the site of the irritation, inflaming the tissue to eliminate the alien intruder. The innate immune system then goes on to take care of the further work to be done. When we have a simpler damage than cancer, for instance, like cutting ourselves with a kitchen knife, the immune systems senses the wound as a hole in our body that has to be filled in.

Dr. Rakoff-Nahoum explains that when inflammation can't end chronic irritation inside the body, the immune system interprets the inflamed area as a wound to be filled in, and signals cells to proliferate. Some of the proliferating cells may mutate and form a tumor. We often think we have cancer because our immune system has failed, but when tumors are examined under a microscope, many kinds of immune system cells are found inside them, creating inflammation and cell proliferation.[10]

Carrots stop inflammation and may slow down or even stop the immune system's mistaken call for growth factors, restoring the healthy community of cells. In the anti-cancer game, chemotherapy and radiation are like angry coaches who, not liking the way the game is going, get out their guns and massacre the players. In contrast, carrots' epigenetic solution to cancer re-educates the players to work together differently.

Seven: Apoptosis and Necrosis

The means carrots use to cure cancer aren't fully understood, but they are clearly superior to those of chemotherapy and radiation. Carrots do no harm to the body; they're cheap, and they're available almost everywhere in the world. If you choose chemotherapy and radiation, it's very much worthwhile to drink carrot juice as well, to increase their effectiveness. The faster chemo and radiation work, the less damage they'll do your body. The longer you use them, the less effective and more damaging they become. Here are some reasons why.

Cancer occurs when cell signaling goes wrong. Attacking cancer, chemotherapy and radiation both assault the immune system. They kill the rapidly growing red and white blood cells forming in the bone marrow. The death of the red blood cells creates anemia. With fewer red blood cells, less oxygen is available to aid in killing cancer cells. Having too few white blood cells, a condition called neutropenia, the immune system can't defend against infection. Anemia makes people weak and fatigued; neutropenia puts them at risk of fatal infections.

There are about 70 trillion cells inside an adult human body. Every second a million old cells die and a million new ones are born. There are two main ways the body kills old, damaged or cancerous cells. The first is apoptosis. The word comes from the ancient Greek, in which it was used to describe the kind of death that comes to a browning leaf in autumn, falling from a tree. Apoptosis is a gentle programmed death in which the cell disintegrates within its own membrane as proteins called caspases enter it to take it apart from inside. No damage from the break-up goes into the bloodstream to cause inflammation. This is the way carrots destroy cancer cells—by apoptosis, which doesn't damage surrounding normal cells.

The second form of cell death is necrosis, another word from the Greek that means "killed thing, dead thing." In necrosis, cells are blasted open and their contents spill into the bloodstream. One scientist has compared an apoptotic death to a suicide—and necrotic death to a train wreck. If you are interested in seeing what necrosis looks like, use an internet browser and type in "necrosis" and "images."

Chemotherapy poisons rapidly dividing cells and damages their DNA. Once damaged, lots of them break down and die—but some don't. Many cancer cells are able to tolerate the chemo attack, repel it, evolve, and stay alive. In contrast, carrots and other natural cures restore natural cell regulation systems in the body, re-sensitizing cells to chemical messages that tell them to die apoptotically.

Chemotherapy and radiation cause some apoptosis, but more often they cause necrosis. Necrosis can be fatal, not just to collapsing individual cells, but to our whole body. When cells die too fast through necrosis, a tremendous mass of dead cell material is sent to the kidneys, overwhelming their capacity to purify the blood.

This overkill is called Tumor Lysis Syndrome. According to the Journal of the American Society of Nephrology, "The massive death of tumor cells can ironically trigger a condition [Tumor Lysis Syndrome] that may itself be fatal to cancer patients, and it occurs in more than 20% of patients with certain cancer types." It happens to nearly 10% of patients who are treated within a week of diagnosis of a new cancer; and it's much more likely to cause death in the very first session of chemo treatment than at any other time.[1]

Chemo- or radiation-caused necrosis may continue months or years after your treatment is finished— attacking healthy cells long after the cancerous cells are gone. Continued necrosis from chemotherapy or radiation can weaken heart muscle and cause heart attacks.

Follow up of close to 20,000 women with breast cancer revealed that radiation therapy reduced the annual mortality from breast cancer by 13%—but increased the annual mortality rate from circulatory problems by

21%—mostly from damage to the heart. Radiation made the survival statistics for cancer look good, while worsening those for heart conditions. The "progress" that lowered total cancer deaths came because women died from heart attacks instead.[2]

During and after chemotherapy, necrosis kills healthy brain cells. For decades, women were told that "chemo brain," the distracted minds and memory loss they suffered after chemotherapy for breast cancer, was "all in their heads"—just natural depression and worry about having cancer. Then, in 2006, Dr. Mark Noble of the University of Rochester Medical Center discovered that in 80% of the women who accept chemotherapy for breast cancer, "chemo brain" is real and organic. Chemotherapy attacks dividing cells in the brain that are meant to hold new memories. The longer and more intense the chemo, the more brain damage. Dr. Noble and his team found that three chemotherapy drugs were more toxic[3] to healthy brain cells than to the cancer they were supposed to treat.

Chemotherapy and radiation cause necrosis. Necrosis creates inflammation. Inflammation stimulates growth factors to create more cancer cells and form new blood vessels to bring them food. A recent study showed that when chemotherapy and radiation attack cancer, they leave behind necrotic cell fragments that the body can't clean up. These chemo- and radiation-caused fragments promote the spread of cancer[4] to distant sites in the body.

Chemotherapy sometimes causes apoptosis, which would be a good thing—except the apoptosis from chemo can include a step called autophagy—from the Greek words "auto" (self), and "phagein" (to eat). Apoptotic cancerous cells can become zombies. Expelling parts of themselves while dying, they can simultaneously "eat" these fragments and use them as a source of energy to bring themselves back to life.[5]

Some researchers see an advantage to necrotic death: when cancer cells treated with chemotherapy or radiation resist apoptosis, necrosis can still destroy them, and continue killing them after treatment's over. The problem is that necrosis doesn't stop with killing only cancer cells. It also kills useful healthy cells.

In one particularly grueling case of cure by necrosis, chemotherapy and whole brain radiation eliminated a woman's brain tumors. However, after her treatment ended, her healthy brain cells continued to die. Her husband, describing her gradual mental deterioration over years, concluded "Believe me, a slow, arduous, neurological death is not preferable to a cancerous one."

Eight: Caution and Chemotherapy

In my experience and that of many people I've talked to, doctors offer chemotherapy almost to the bitter end of the cancer journey—and enthusiastically, with far too little discussion of the damage it can cause, the reasons it can fail, and the doubts about its statistical claims to success.

The most dubious offer from oncologists is palliative chemotherapy—the chemo that can't cure, but is intended to shrink tumors and extend life. Many patients don't ask how long, on average, their life might be extended—this is usually a matter of only a few months, painful news oncologists don't necessarily share with patients unless they're asked. In England, a study recorded patient-doctor discussions of palliative chemotherapy and concluded: "Most patients are not given clear information about the survival benefit of palliative chemotherapy..."

Palliative chemotherapy uses drugs the same as or similar to those of "adjuvant" chemotherapy and causes similar side effects. Not knowing this, patients may make decisions they wouldn't make if they were fully informed. The English study points out that there's a very low survival benefit for palliative treatment and sometimes the side effects shorten lives.[1]

Dictionaries define a "palliative treatment" as one that doesn't attack the cause of a disease, but is rather intended to relieve pain. In theory, shrinking a tumor should lessen suffering. However, in another English study, 43% of mostly incurable patients suffered toxicity and pain from the palliative chemo treatments.[2] One in four died from the effects of chemotherapy rather than from the cancer itself.

In 2012, the *New York Times* reported on a study of cancer and pain published in *Journal of Clinical Oncology*.

> Researchers surveyed more than 3,000 cancer patients and found that nearly two-thirds said they were in pain or receiving pain medications. Roughly a third felt they needed more painkillers to fully treat their symptoms. A month after the patients saw their oncologists, the researchers again asked the patients about their pain. Instead of showing improvement, the percentage of patients who continued to be in pain remained unchanged. The findings are a sobering echo of research from nearly two decades ago that revealed that more than 40% of cancer patients did not receive adequate treatment for their pain. Nearly a third of cancer specialists waited until

the patient was only months away from death before offering maximum pain control.[3]

Oncologists convince patients of the importance of "tumor response" (shrinkage) as the measure of successful treatment, even though they know that usually chemotherapy and radiation shrink tumors only temporarily and a patient soon requires another, less effective, course of chemotherapy—"second line" or "third line" chemotherapy with different drugs.

Patients' comments online about chemotherapy and new post-chemotherapy drugs are full of reports of debilitating effects; they usually conclude, saying, "But my tumor has shrunk" or "But I'm still alive, and that's the main thing." Though patients hope for a cure, they have been taught not to expect one—to think instead about "five-year overall survival" and to resign themselves to the possibility that five years later they may only be hanging on to life by a thread, undergoing more damaging treatments.

Standard treatments rarely cure cancer. Biopsies and surgeries can cause metastases. Chemotherapy and radiation are carcinogenic and may stimulate a return of cancer that's resistant to treatment, or a new cancer that comes many years later.[4] Chemotherapy is poisonous. Our cells have built-in protections against poisons. Every cell, cancerous or normal, has a pump inside it that expels chemotherapeutic drugs, sending them back to the bloodstream and out of the body. These pumps become ever more efficient as chemo treatments continue.[5]

Many cancer researchers devote themselves to studying the problems of radiation resistance and chemo-resistance. Their findings are discouraging.

When radiation or chemotherapy attacks cancer cells, the most vulnerable cells die rapidly and tumors are reduced. Unfortunately, the tougher tumor cells that survive usually become even stronger and repopulate the tumor. Because the treatments are so hard on normal cells, the patient needs breaks from treatment. During those breaks, the cancer doesn't rest, it grows. To get "the best outcome" for patients, at least 85% of the ideal recommended chemotherapy doses are necessary,[6] but in many cases it's impossible to give that much.

Cancer industry statistics indicate that people who take chemotherapy and radiation live longer than those who refuse them. But is that true? People who die before completing radiation or chemotherapy treatment for cancer aren't included in the statistics on the disease. Exclusion is fair enough when these patients got hit by a bus on the way to a chemo session. After all, in that case it's not the fault of treatment that they didn't reach five-year survival. But if they died as a consequence of treatment, cancer statistics should reflect that fact, and they don't. Most people who get fatal illnesses from cancer treatments have their cause of death recorded as[7] "pneumonia" or "cardiac arrest" among others, rather than as "consequence of cancer treatment." They might have lived longer—and more happily—minus their treatments.

Cancer patients take on grueling chemo or radiation

because the official statistics about a particular drug seem to promise a longer life. An oncologist will report that in a major study, the group who took it lived two years longer than those took no drug; or that they lived two and a half months longer than those who took a competing product. The statistics rarely include adequate information on quality of life.

Most clinical trials on individual drugs are financed by drug companies who sell them. Given the tremendous profits to be made with a new cancer drug, it isn't surprising that clinical trial results are often fabricated. In her book, *The Truth about Drug Companies: How They Deceive Us and What To Do About It*, Dr. Marcia Angell, former editor of the *New England Journal of Medicine*, says, "Trials can be rigged in a dozen ways[8], and it happens all the time." In a recent article she wrote:

> Most doctors take money or gifts from drug companies in one way or another. Many are paid consultants, speakers at company-sponsored meetings, ghost-authors of papers written by drug companies or their agents, and ostensible "researchers" whose contribution often consists merely of putting their patients on a drug and transmitting some token information to the company. Still more doctors are recipients of free meals and other out-and-out gifts. In addition, drug companies subsidize most meetings of professional organizations and most of the continuing medical education needed by doctors to maintain their state licenses.

No one knows the total amount provided by drug companies to physicians, but I estimate from the annual reports of the top nine US drug companies that it comes to tens of billions of dollars a year. By such means, the pharmaceutical industry has gained enormous control over how doctors evaluate and use its own products. Its extensive ties to physicians, particularly senior faculty at prestigious medical schools, affect the results of research, the way medicine is practiced, and even the definition of what constitutes a disease.[9]

A chemotherapy drug or radiation in some circumstances may be vital for your survival. But it's a good idea to investigate before you buy.

Nine: Carrot Liberation

Oncologists can tell the truth yet mislead by omission—leaving out a full picture of a treatment's likelihood of long-term success or failure, and its effects. Because of these omissions, patients may consent to treatments they would otherwise reject. The luteolin in carrots could liberate them from the side effects of two very common drugs.

Liberation from Avastin

As discussed in Chapter Six, tumors can grow large only if they can stimulate angiogenesis—the formation of new blood vessels to bring them food. Avastin, currently the best-selling drug in the world, was developed to stop tumor angiogenesis and is usually prescribed for it. Avastin costs up to $100,000 a year per patient in the US.[1] Even patients with insurance can be financially devastated by the out-of-pocket costs for this drug.

On average, Avastin extends cancer patients' lives by only two months. It prevents tumor angiogenesis, but it also prevents healthy blood vessels from repairing themselves. Avastin can open holes in the intestines and the nose, prevent surgery sites from healing, and damage the circulatory system.[2] The *Harvard Heart Letter* places Avastin near the top of the list of new drugs causing damage to the heart.[3]

In-vitro and animal experiments show that luteolin stops angiogenesis.[4] Wouldn't it be much less risky—and cheaper—for cancer patients to prevent angiogenesis by drinking luteolin-rich carrot juice?

Liberation from Tamoxifen

30% of breast cancer survivors have a recurrence of cancer; 70% don't.[5] Oncologists don't know which patients are among the endangered 30% and which are among the safe 70%. To prevent new breast cancer, they normally prescribe all their breast cancer survivors a grueling five-year or ten-year course of Tamoxifen. Tamoxifen is an estrogen-blocking drug. In some cases, estrogen getting to the breast can stimulate cell proliferation. Oncologists believe that preventing estrogen from getting to the breast will help block a cancer recurrence.

However, a healthy body needs estrogen.[6] Like Avastin, Tamoxifen goes too far.

Users of Tamoxifen report difficulty thinking. In a 2004 study comparing three groups of women—those who used Tamoxifen, those who used supplemental estrogen, and those who used neither—the Tamoxifen users had the lowest scores on word memory tests and lower metabolism in two areas of the brain.[7] Entirely blocking estrogen to the breast for five years or ten years has many bad consequences. Tamoxifen and its kindred drugs are horrific for many users. At the website *askapatient.com*, one woman reported Tamoxifen's effects on her life. "Leg cramps at night; joints hurting on waking every morning: nausea at the 2-3 week mark; muscle fatigue after short period of exercise; depression, crying daily, short temper. Not sure that I, or my family, can put up with these side-effects long term. Might extend my likelihood of the cancer not coming back, but at what personal price?"

A study by Mark Noble of the University of Rochester Medical Center found that with two days of Tamoxifen exposure at the level patients use, 75% of a certain kind of brain cell died—cells essential for making the insulating sheaths required for nerves to work properly.[8]

A 2009 article in *Natural News* reports on a study showing that Tamoxifen, while decreasing risk for one kind of breast cancer, puts women in danger of a second, far more dangerous type of breast cancer.[9] Breast cancer patients prescribed Femara, Arimidex, Zometa and other substitutes for Tamoxifen also suffer bad effects.[10]

Luteolin binds to estrogen receptors in the breast more strongly than Tamoxifen. It inhibits cell proliferation there without doing any damage to health.[11] If oncologists were aware that long-term use of

Tamoxifen creates much more serious cancer, and that luteolin prevents cancer cell proliferation without doing harm, wouldn't they would stop prescribing women Tamoxifen and prescribe either luteolin, or just carrots, instead?

Before accepting a prescription of Avastin, Tamoxifen or one of the Tamoxifen substitutes, people should ask their doctors for the evidence that these drugs prevent cancer any better than carrot juice.

Ten: Puzzles of Profitability

Why don't oncologists prescribe carrot juice at $15 a week to prevent angiogenesis, instead of sometimes fatal Avastin at $100,000 a year?

Why don't oncologists prescribe carrot juice to prevent a return of breast cancer, when the luteolin in it works so well? Why, when Tamoxifen stimulates new, more serious breast cancers, do oncologists recommend five or ten years of it "just in case," so women can be "safe"?

Probably they've never heard of luteolin. Perhaps from habit they prescribe what drug salespeople suggest and what standard oncology journals advertise.

It's in oncologists' financial interest to prescribe expensive drugs, and certainly that eases their way into believing in them.[1] In the USA, as of 2013 the average oncologist's annual salary was $265,723, and the highest paid among them received $685,000 per year.

A large part of a U.S. oncologist's income—often well over half—derives from the sale of chemotherapy drugs. A 2011 article from the *New England Journal of Medicine* explained:

> Unlike other drugs, chemotherapeutics are bought and sold in the doctor's office—a practice that originated 40 years ago, when only oncologists would handle such toxic substances and the drugs were relatively cheap. A business model evolved in which oncologists bought low and sold high to support their practice and maximize financial margins. Oncologists buy drugs from wholesalers, mark them up, and sell them to patients (or insurers) in the office. Since medical oncology is a cognitive specialty lacking associated procedures, without drug sales, oncologists' salaries would be lower than geriatricians'. In recent decades, oncology-drug prices have skyrocketed, and today more than half the revenue of an oncology office may come from chemotherapy sales.
>
> Before 2003, Medicare reimbursed oncologists 95% of the average wholesale price—an unregulated price set by manufacturers—whereas oncologists paid 66 to 88% of that price and thus received $1.6 billion annually in over-payments. To blunt unsustainable cost increases, the Medicare Modernization Act mandated that the Centers for Medicare and Medicaid Services (CMS) set reimbursement at the average sales price plus a 6% markup to cover practice costs. This policy has reduced not only drug payments but also demand for generics. In some

cases, the reimbursement is less than the cost of administration. For instance, the price of a vial of carboplatin has fallen from $125 to $3.50, making the 6% payment trivial. So some oncologists switched to higher-margin brand-name drugs. Why use paclitaxel (and receive 6% of $312) when you can use Abraxane (for 6% of $5,824)?[2]

If you were an oncologist, would you prescribe carrots and get no commission whatsoever, when you can prescribe Avastin and get 6% of a hundred thousand dollars a year?

If as a cancer patient, you discover that your oncologist's prescription of Avastin or Abraxane is going to cost you $10,000, you might explain to your oncologist that you can't afford it. He or she can probably find a cheaper substitute.

Studies have shown that gratitude, nice meals, and favors from drug companies play a major role in oncologists' prescriptions. When polled on this subject, oncologists all say their colleagues are swayed by these promotional efforts, but that they themselves are not.[3]

Dr. John R. Lee, M.D., author of *What Your Doctor May Not Tell You About Breast Cancer*, has comments applicable to the medical profession's approach to all cancers:

> The politics of physician attitudes that don't support healing, medical research, and media information on breast cancer are disheartening, because they're largely controlled by large drug companies with one

agenda: Sell more drugs. At the root of physician beliefs and attitudes about breast cancer treatment is the fact that the pharmaceutical industry now powerfully influences both medical education and research. A recent Journal of the American Medical Association (JAMA) reported that 31% of medical school funding comes from governmental and pharmaceutical grants; we think this is a gross underestimate.

In addition, drug company money is the driving force behind medical research, with a profound influence on the research that's chosen. For example, if a drug that has the potential to be patented is competing for funding with a drug that can't be patented because it's found in nature, there's no contest. The patent drug wins, even if the drug found in nature might be the biggest breakthrough since penicillin.[4]

Oncologists may not know much about natural ingredients and their effect on cancer, but the big drug companies do know; they're very interested in patenting components that can be isolated from them. As the *Journal of Nutrition* reports, isolated ingredients don't heal as effectively as whole foods; but drug companies can't sell whole foods or entirely natural products. That's why they promote cancer-stimulating progestin for hormone replacement therapy, rather than also available natural progesterone. One day, decades in the future, drug companies will make ingeniously altered compounds from carrots into highly promoted capsules or creams. They may or not be good for you, but they'll definitely carry a high price. It's better not to wait.

Right now you can drink carrot juice and learn its benefits for yourself.

Eleven: Making Decisions

INTERVIEW YOURSELF

Most oncologists justify conventional treatments old and new, arguing that even though they often don't work, there's nothing else that will. They admit that chemo and radiation can cause your body long-term permanent damage or even a new cancer years in the future, but, they say, you should worry about today: you are better off stopping your present cancer than worrying about a cancer you may get months or years later. Now the clock is ticking, chemo and radiation are waiting, and your oncologist is ready with a treatment plan for you.

Is the moment of diagnosis really an emergency? Usually not. Most likely your cancer has been growing a long time and isn't about to kill you within hours. Probably you have time to mull things over for a few days or longer and investigate for yourself any treatment proposed for you before you accept it. You will have many questions when you interview your doctor. But first, you would be wise to interview yourself.

Confronted with the chilling statistics about cancer, our first impulse may be to accept every treatment our doctors recommend and be one of the exceptions, one of the lucky patients who will be cured. But if our determination to survive is mostly panic—a fear of our mortality—our first reaction can prevent us from thinking clearly.

Years ago, I came across a quote from the English author, Somerset Maugham, that changed me and many of my decisions. Maugham said, "It is a funny thing about life; if you refuse to accept anything but the best, you very often get it."

When I got cancer, I wanted the best—not three more years of life, not four years of treatments and a new cancer two years later. I wanted a cure. If I couldn't have the best, I was ready to accept death. I don't say this is the right choice for others. Much about cancer depends on one's individual character and life circumstances, and particularly, one's age. But often, when we ensnare ourselves in accepting less than what we really want, we lose our chances for the best.

Facing the reality of death squarely can do a lot to clarify who we most deeply are, what we want from life and how we want to live the time left to us.

When you get a diagnosis of cancer, before you interview your doctors, interview yourself. Resolve that you'll deal with your cancer in the way that is the absolute best for you. Refuse to be scared of it, because if you are scared of it, it can defeat you. You can work against it better if you fully accept its dangers. In the U.S. most of us prepare for everything in life but death. But to live our best, we need to recognize and prepare for that final challenge.

As soon as you're diagnosed with cancer, and ideally, long before, you can prepare a living will, an advance directive and, in some U.S. states, a POLST order.[1] Name a legal health care proxy who will make health decisions for you if you can't. Keep these papers in a place that's easy to get to, and tell those you care about where the papers are. Make sure your loved ones know how much treatment you want; any treatments you definitely don't want; and when, if the cancer can't be stopped, you want to end conventional treatment. (A helpful new foundation set up to make it easier for you to explore your values and share them with your family is called The Conversation Project.)[2] If you don't make things clear to your family, the time may come when you can't speak for yourself; and the bitter disagreements among your loved ones about what you really want could divide them for life.

Your evaluation of standard treatments will depend on your age. If you're thirty years old with a potentially fatal cancer and you risk an extreme treatment that makes you very sick, but eliminates cancer, you may gain 45 years more of life. You undergo major risks for potentially a big payoff. If you're seventy years old and have the same treatment, your risk of treatment complications leaving you disabled is much greater than for the thirty-year-old. Moreover, the big jackpot—45 probable years of further life, is not available to you.

At seventy, life expectancy is about ten years. Suppose you succeed in defeating cancer at 70 and lowering your risk of its return to near zero, but treatment also reduced your quality of life to near zero and you soon die of pneumonia. What will your sacrifices for cancer treatment have accomplished?

At any age, when you interview yourself, ask how much treatment you want. How much are you willing to pay for it in terms of physical suffering and financial cost? Would you want members of your family to mortgage their homes and go into debt to give you every chance to live a little longer, even if your quality of life were gone? Answer these questions while you feel relatively good and have the strength to deal with them. Let everyone important to you know your decisions and put them in writing. Look into the laws of your state to find out what documents you need to make your health care choices medically and legally binding.

USING THE INTERNET FOR RESEARCH

Making the decision to first try "carrots only" can radically simplify your cancer treatment considerations, probably saving you many thousands of dollars, and possibly curing you. But whatever cancer treatment interests you, including carrots, research it yourself. This is how.

Your first concern will probably be to find out how standard cancer survival statistics predict your length of life. To get search for that information, enter as your search term the kind and stage of your cancer, and the words "overall survival"—the figure that includes people who haven't died from cancer or any other cause in the listed time-frame. When you read the results, remember that they are based on almost entirely on people who have accepted surgery, chemotherapy and radiation as their treatments, and who probably weren't advised to make any dietary improvements in response to their cancer. With the cancer education this book is giving you, you have a good chance for a better outcome than statistics show.

Your next concern may be to investigate alternative treatments. If you are interested in using acai berries to cure your cancer, type in "acai berries" and "cancer fraud" on an internet search. Then, "acai berries" and "cancer cure." Evaluate what you read for and against a given treatment. To get the most recent research first, add a date, like "2013" or "2014" to your inquiry. Using Google, you can enter up to 32 words per search.

Perhaps you think of having "Slammer" electromagnetic treatments from Sara Smith (a fictitious treatment from a healer whose name I've just invented). You hear about Sara from a friend and want to know more about her. Look up "Sara Smith" with the words "Slammer" "cancer treatment" and "complaints" or "fraud." Then look Sara up again with the word "cure." If you see a website that tells you she has a Ph.D. in Biochemistry from the University of California, check on her credentials. Google her name with the words "Sara Smith" and "Ph.D." and "University of California." If you read that she has a diploma from "Slammer Technology School," Google "Slammer Technology School" and "cancer cure," then Google "Slammer Technology" and "complaints" or "fraud." (You can also do your research on Sara's treatment the old-fashioned way: ask Sara for references, with phone numbers, so you can talk to others she's treated. Ask for some referrals to people who consulted her less recently, so you can be sure that you're hearing about lasting results, not just hope and the placebo effect. Talking to her clients, ask for detailed description of treatments—not just a "Sara's great!" response. When did the person see her, and for how long? What's the state of the cancer now?)

If you get cancer, probably your primary care doctor will refer you to cancer specialists at a hospital near you. If you have worries about hospital quality, it can help to talk to friends about their experiences in the one you've been referred to. You can also use the internet to type in a hospital name and the words "patient reviews." In the U.S., an excellent way to learn about their quality is to use a national website for nurses, allnurses.com, where nurses advise each other on working conditions in specific hospitals. A hospital that nurses say is understaffed and under-equipped is one for you to avoid.

Some corporate hospital chains are ruthless in squeezing every possible dollar from patients, and doctors must comply with those methods or lose their jobs. One, Health Management Associates, has been sued by the U.S. Department of Justice for false Medicare reimbursement claims. To increase its income, HMA forced its doctors to admit Medicare- insured people to its hospitals when they were perfectly healthy. Although the Justice Department has fined HMA very heavily, its profits are so big that the fines become just a minor cost of doing business.[3] Community Health Systems, an even bigger chain, has now bought HMA.

To learn about oncologists, check with friends and also the internet to research their reputations. Let's say you want to learn about Wallace Wellness, M.D., the oncologist you've just consulted. Has anyone brought a lawsuit against him for medical negligence? Many doctors get sued unfairly—but it wouldn't hurt to do an internet search of his name with the words "patient reviews" "medical negligence," "complaints" or maybe "litigation."

If you suspect that doctors may be biased because they receive income from drug companies, you can look them up through ProPublica, an organization for journalism in the public interest. I looked up my Portland, Oregon oncologist and surgeon, and found out they were not accepting such payments. That increased my faith in them.

To find out about side effects of individual drugs, go to websites which list them. If, for example, your doctor recommends Cisplatin, search the drug by name with the words "price" and "side effects." You will find that its side effects can be pretty nasty, and can range from ringing in the ears to total deafness, a complete loss of balance and inability to walk. Then you might look up "percentage with loss of balance" or whatever other percentages concern you. Following that search, it would be useful to look up together, your kind of cancer, and "alternatives to Cisplatin." You'll find what might be prescribed as alternative drugs, and their side effects. Askapatient.com, webMD.com. drugs.com, rx.com, and other sites provide detailed patient reports on their experiences with cancer drugs. It's true that usually people who have a worse, or better than usual, response to a drug, are the ones who comment. But don't discount the commenters: you could respond to a treatment just as they have.

For an estimate of how many people are damaged by a particular treatment, look up clinical studies of particular drugs by name, with the name of the drug, the words "grade of toxicity" and "clinical studies." Oncology research grading of drug toxicity goes from 1 (no side effects) to 5 (death). If you see many ratings of 3 and above, you are probably looking at a drug that might be fatal for you. Often after a drug is approved on the basis of the manufacturer's clinical trial, a later independent study shows a higher level of toxicity than the earlier trials.

Some scientific journals charge to view their articles. Both public and university libraries subscribe to many journals and offer readers free access to them. If you do your research in these libraries, you won't have to pay to read studies that interest you.

If you aren't strong enough or well enough or computer savvy enough to do this kind of research for yourself, have a friend do it for you.

INTERVIEW YOUR DOCTOR

With the sudden blow of a cancer diagnosis, you're guaranteed to forget, misremember, or misinterpret something your doctors say. Therefore, don't see your cancer physicians alone. Always take a family member or friend to your appointments. Choose somebody who stays cool and can take notes. Ask the doctor to explain any words you don't understand and spell them, so you can look them up later. Be sure you understand clearly the risks of treatments proposed for you. Read the fine print on reports of your cancer, and look up the definitions of any unfamiliar words. Take a digital recorder to each meeting with your doctors and listen to the whole conversation later to be sure you get all the details.

If you are determined to try natural treatments first, at your initial appointment make that clear to the oncologist. Ask if in your circumstances you can afford to wait eight weeks before turning to conventional treatment. If your oncologist is entirely opposed to natural treatments, ask to be referred to an oncologist with an interest in them. You need an oncologist who can support and guide you, or at least respect your choice and listen. Providing an oncologist information about cancer-related studies of luteolin, falcarinol, and carrots might help gain professional support for your choice.

As a patient, you give your informed consent to treatment. That doesn't mean just a casual "Sign here." The legal requirement for your informed consent exists to protect you. When you are informed, you have learned the purpose of the proposed treatment, and its record of success. You should understand all its side effects—how frequently they occur, how severe they can be and how long they might last. How many patients drop the treatment rather than completing it? You should be told the length of treatment, and how it compares to alternatives, including doing nothing.

If you consider chemo or radiation, ask about their effect on your appetite. As mentioned earlier, 80% of cancer patients suffer malnutrition during treatment.[4] Just at the time people vitally need maximum nutrition, they often don't want to eat, or can't. Chemo usually causes nausea, a sour metallic taste to food, and lack of appetite. Radiation can burn your throat so badly that you'll have to be hospitalized and fed intravenously. According to the National Cancer Institute, 20% to 40% of cancer patients die from causes related to malnutrition, not from the cancer itself.

Dr. Kevin Block, M.D., Medical Director of the Block Center for Integrative Cancer Treatment, points out that "Unfortunately, conventional medical advice suggesting a patient eat whatever they want, can actually feed the patient's cancer, promote their malnutrition, and contribute to the patient's inability to tolerate treatment."

If you decide to use conventional treatments, you can make them work better by drinking carrot juice as you take them—preferably, no less than five cups of fresh carrot juice daily. The effects of carrots can only be good for you. Because carrots are anti-inflammatory, even if they don't cure your cancer, they will help you feel better. If later you decide you no longer need or want them, you'll have lost nothing on account of them—not your hair, your memory or your job.

Tell your doctor you must have adequate pain medication if your illness gets worse, and get details about how that will be arranged. The National Cancer Institute provides detailed information about kinds of pain control, its cost, and insurance coverage. To prevent sales of painkillers to addicts, the US Drug Enforcement Agency tracks doctors' prescriptions. To avoid problems with the DEA, among other reasons, doctors often under-prescribe painkillers to patients who need them. Those who demand better pain control will get it, but those who don't, may not.[5]

Give yourself time to make your decision or to seek a second opinion or a third opinion. If information you get is contradictory and confusing, ask enough questions to clarify it. If you feel your doctor is evasive, is hustling you or is more of a salesman than a doctor, find another. You have a right to refuse any treatment that you believe will damage you. Make sure your doctor can justify clearly the benefits of whatever treatments he or she proposes. What's the evidence for them?

If your oncologist quotes statistics from clinical studies, ask how the study group compares to you. Were they your age? Are you likely to have an outcome like theirs? You might ask your oncologist how frequently in his or her experience, your kind of cancer responds to treatment and is actually cured, without having a return of cancer. If you get discouraging information or none, it may be time for you to choose a natural treatment. Most attention in cancer statistics is given to five-year survival, but you can also ask about two-year, three-year or ten-year survival figures.

There are some important terms to differentiate when you ask your oncologist about these statistics. For instance, "absolute survival" is the percentage of people with a particular cancer who five years later are still alive, with or without cancer and with or without quality of life. What is likely to concern you more than "absolute survival" is your chance of being cancer free in five years. That's "disease-free survival." You may want to ask your oncologist, "If I complete the course of treatment you propose, what is my chance for 'five year disease-free survival'?" (Being "Disease free" indicates you are free of cancer, not of other diseases, including ones cancer treatment may have caused. You can ask about "over-all" survival—that's your chance of overcoming all causes of death for a given period.)

You may also want to ask about a comparative number, your "five-year relative survival." 'Relative survival' is the term used to compare a cancer patient's chances for being alive in a certain number of years, with cancer, or cancer free, to the average 5-year survival percentage of cancer-free people your age.

If you are elderly, your oncologist may say, "If you take the treatment, statistics show that your five-year relative survival is 90%." This sounds very encouraging only because your comparison population without cancer now has a shorter life expectancy. The 90% figure could mean, for instance, that those who don't have cancer have a 30% chance of being alive five years from now, and you, if you take the proposed chemo or radiation, have a 27% chance of being alive in five years. Those who are cancer-free are only 3% more likely to be alive five years from now. Is it worth taking treatment for a 3% improvement in your life expectancy?

A study about mathematically evaluating risks versus benefits of cancer treatment concluded:

> Because older patients have many competing risks for death, the absolute effect of a new diagnosis on life expectancy is often relatively small. Consequently, the potential gain in survival even from perfect therapy may also be small. Moreover, no therapy is perfect, and the risks of therapy often increase with age. In the elderly, the combination of a high burden of competing risks and high rates of treatment-related complications conspires to reduce the net benefit of numerous interventions. We conclude that, compared with younger patients, the elderly should request only the more clearly effective treatments and should be willing to tolerate fewer associated complications before they agree to initiate therapy.[6]

Don't get so hooked on anyone's promises for a better future with a specific treatment that you won't give it up if it ravages your body and your life. Using meditation and positive visualization techniques can help keep you oriented to your hopes and best self. No matter your diagnosis, you can resolve to live every moment as well as you possibly can.

CANCER CARE AND YOUR WALLET

Most U.S. health care organizations, even supposedly non-profit institutions, exist to make a profit. U.S. health care has become big business—too big. An organization called *StrikeDebt* describes the situation this way: "Private health care enriches a few—insurance companies, private equity firms, pharmaceutical companies, debt collectors, and global investors—at the expense of everyone else."[7]

Like many other industries, U.S. health care works hard to develop more and more products to increase its sales and more persuasive means of selling them. Not all its products are worth buying. Interviewed recently, Dr. Angelo Volandes of Harvard Medical School said, "In the healthcare debate, we've heard a lot about useless care, wasteful care, futile care. What we…have been struggling with is unwanted care. That's far more concerning. That's not avoidable care. That's *wrongful* care. I think that's the most urgent issue facing America today, is people getting medical interventions that, if they were more informed, they would not want. It happens all the time."[8]

Dr. Otis Brawley, Vice President of the American Cancer Society and author of *How We Do Harm: A Doctor Breaks Ranks about Being Sick in America*, says the U.S. healthcare system is "subtly corrupt." It needs to be transformed, he says, and only an informed public—that's you and me—can do it. In a speech, he told science journalists:

> We need to understand and appreciate science. We're not going to have improvements in our healthcare

system until the mass population demands that doctors appreciate science, justify their recommendations and justify their decisions. We need the skeptical, educated consumer. We need people who consume medicine to think about health care the same way they think about buying a television set at a Best Buy.[9]

Medical treatments cause 62% of personal bankruptcies in the U.S.[10] Most people bankrupted by medical care are average Americans—with medical insurance. Even with the Affordable Care Act, most "affordable" insurance carries high deductibles: people go deeply into debt to pay for uncovered costs of treatment. If, as a result of illness they can't work and lose their jobs, they fall even more disastrously into debt. In fact, half of all home foreclosures in the U.S. are the result of medical debt.[11]

The financial pressures of cancer treatment, hospitalizations, drugs, travel to faraway cancer centers, hotels for family members, and time missed from work can cause major stress. Researchers have found that stress causes cancer to metastasize.[12] I would never recommend the carrot treatment as simply a cost-saving measure; but it's obvious that more carrots and less chemo could mean much less stress for you.

USA Today, in the article "Boomers Face Crisis in Cancer Care" (September 2013) notes that of 13 cancer treatments approved by the Food and Drug Administration in 2012, only one was proven to extend survival by more than a median of six months.[13] The drugs all cost more than $5,900 per month.

When you talk to your oncologist, ask what your out-of-pocket costs will be for any drug proposed, and explain that the cost of treatment is very important to you and a major consideration in choosing a hospital. Let your doctors know from the beginning that you don't want to be burdened with debt from unnecessary treatments or those of questionable value.

Get complete information about costs, whether you're buying mistletoe off the internet, seeing a naturopath, or choosing an oncologist. Your oncologist might assume there's no harm in prescribing you high-cost drugs—after all, the bill is going to your insurance company, not to you. But if you explain that you can't afford uncovered charges and that a recommended treatment is far beyond your means, your doctors may find a cheaper alternative.

If you have to take on debt to pay for treatment, don't put it on your credit card. Things go wrong and you may not be able to pay: interest charges and penalties for late payment can bankrupt you. It's better to make a payment plan with the hospital. Ask for all bills to be itemized. Separate doctors' bills from hospital bills. Make sure you're not double-billed. Keep a dated, detailed record of appointments, tests and treatments and when you've paid for them.

Better hospitals usually have a financial officer whose job is to help you find ways to lower your costs. Nonprofit hospitals must comply with new IRS rulings that offer you some protection when they deal with your medical debt. If you feel that a hospital is more interested in billing you than helping you, look for a different hospital.

WHEN CHEMO CAN'T CURE CANCER

In 2013, a presenter at an American Society of Clinical Oncology Symposium warned, "Patients receiving chemotherapy solely for palliative intent have a high risk of chemotherapy-related hospitalization, defeating the goal of the care and increasing healthcare costs."[14]

If palliative chemotherapy can extend your life only briefly, painfully, and very expensively, you may do better treating yourself with carrot juice. If you have savings, use them for a marvelous trip you've always wanted to make, or invest them in your children's or grandchildren's education.

Why, when oncologists tell patients that their cancers are incurable by chemotherapy, do patients choose more chemotherapy?

Maybe it's because they're too emotionally devastated to absorb the news, or maybe it's because their doctors don't speak to them clearly enough. A recent study showed that 75% of cancer patients, told that more chemotherapy and radiation can't cure their cancer, believe their doctors have said the opposite.[15]

Patients who are incurable by radiation and chemotherapy mostly want to spend their remaining months or years at home, with family, rather than in hospital from treatment-caused emergencies.

An October 2013 article in *U.S. News*, "Weighing Over-Treatment vs. Ending Treatment" observed, "Half a million Americans die of cancer each year, and far too many of them die in ways they do not want: hospitalized, in an ICU, unaware of loved ones."

A hospice worker, Sandra Allen Nash, commented on the article: "…I see many suffer through course after course of excruciating treatment and I often suspect that if the diagnosis hadn't been made the patient would have actually lived longer and with a much better quality of life. I fear the oncologists will never stop trying to cure that which they know is incurable and almost never give the patient the truth about the consequences of the treatment, or a clear view of their option to enter a hospice and actually live out their days in peace and comfort."[16]

Interviewed on National Public Radio, Dr. Ira Byock, a specialist in cancer and palliative medicine, and the author of *The Best Care Possible*, said many doctors have a difficult time breaking painful news to patients:

> The open secret among clinicians is we really care about the people who are our patients. …That's not unwholesome. …We get close to these people, and I think … aren't clear in their communication. It's wrong. It's not good practice. But in fact, we hate to make people cry. And it sounds funny to say, but in fact I've seen so many good clinicians—oncologists come to mind, but also cardiologists—who are reticent to tell somebody that their disease is incurable.[17]

In some parts of the U.S. many cancer patients wind up getting useless treatments up to the week before their death and die in a hospital in intensive care.[18] In Canada a study shows that almost half of terminal cancer patients die in hospital, although they say they would prefer to die at home.[19] This is more likely to happen to those who choose palliative chemotherapy than to those who decline it.[20] Often it's because their families, refusing to understand that death has become inevitable, won't let them go. Frequently it's because doctors haven't shared their prognoses with patients honestly.[21] We need to realize that eventually, the time comes for everyone to let go.

If you are a cancer patient, pressure can come from friends, family, doctors, the media and even yourself. The best way to manage the crises of cancer is to educate yourself and take time to think before making decisions. Make them only when you've listened to your inner voice —your deepest self, which knows how to guide you beyond fear.

Twelve: Cures and Improvements

To sum up my own cancer adventure: it could have been a lot worse. My oncologist was a caring person, and she was honest in telling me the bad news—that cancer is difficult to treat and that many people don't make their fifth anniversary of diagnosis. But she didn't discuss at all what might have caused my cancer and how I might have prevented it. And she didn't tell me any of the good news. She didn't mention the new findings in epigenetics. She didn't tell me that cancer was a systemic disease of disordered cell signaling, and that perhaps, if normal cell signaling was restored, I could be healed. After I had chosen carrots instead of chemo and eliminated my cancer, she told me that she believes many natural treatments are effective in attacking cancer. But beforehand, she didn't make any inquiries about my diet, or give any suggestions about improving it.

It seems that many oncologists don't know about the

scientific studies on epigenetics, or on carrots, luteolin, falcarinol, and other anti-cancer foods. I think they ought to; and they ought to tell their patients about them. I've also been told in their defense that they aren't allowed to do this: their professional obligation is to recommend only "proven treatments" backed by statistics (no matter how discouraging). I'm told oncologists would risk de-licensing or a lawsuit from any patient who interpreted their mention of diet as a reason to choose carrots over chemotherapy and wound up dissatisfied.

My mother, who grew up in a town of 300 people in the woods of northern Wisconsin at the beginning of the twentieth century, told me about her neighbor, famous "Dr. Top." Dr. Top was visited by thousands of sick people, coming from as far away as Chicago, to take tonics he'd created in his home. My mother said "Dr. Top" was probably not an M.D. at all, and she wasn't sure if his tonics did anybody any good. Soon in the new century, medical "standards of care" and strict medical licensing were developed all over the U.S. to protect people from unlicensed, unregulated, and possibly uneducated healers like Dr. Top.

Eliminating the "Dr. Tops" of the country also protected the medical guild from competition. It has led over time to a rigid system of compartmentalized medical specialties, with heavy penalties for deviating from "proven treatments" and stepping out of one's box onto some other professional's turf. We citizens pay the price now in a very expensive medical system where not being found wrong is much more important than being right.

If somehow oncologists can't talk to all their patients about cancer prevention and the effects of nutrition on cancer, it's up to you and me to do it.

The number of people I've heard from who are using carrots against cancer in a dedicated way are small, but the successes are remarkable.

I cured metastasized colon cancer with carrots, while Ralph Cole defeated squamous cell cancer, Lung, brain, esophageal, breast, prostate, and bladder and pelvic cancers have also responded to the carrot juice treatment. Here are reports from those who've cured themselves of other cancers with carrot juice. (For clarity, I've edited their comments to standardize spelling and grammar.)

Esophageal Cancer:

Case 1

Mark wrote me in January 2014:

My girlfriend was recently diagnosed with a return of cancerous tumors in her throat/lymph nodes area. She had them removed through surgery and radiation two years ago. This time they were wanting to do the same thing. She has been really nervous with thoughts of having to go through it all over again. ... a couple of weeks ago we started her juicing five pounds of carrots a day and I am happy to say that when she went to the surgeon for a consultation, he said from the time of her ultrasound to the recent scan, which was a couple of weeks, the tumors have been "aggressively shrinking".

February 9, 2014 update:

The doctor said that there was no trace of cancer left and that she would not even need radiation. We are both thrilled! Thank you so much for helping to spread this important information about juicing with carrots. Because of caring people like you and Ralph we were able to try something that has done more than we could have hoped for. We are also trying to tell as many people as possible.

Case 2

Maria posted on amazon.com in a review of this book:

Was healed of Lymph node cancer in the throat after juicing five pounds of carrots a day for about a month. Was going to have to have surgery, radiation, and possibly chemo when first diagnosed. I had to go through several months of back and forth testing with the doctors who, not all but most, refused to accept that they were gone without traditional treatment.

Lung Cancer

On November 1, 2013, Jose in Los Angeles, diagnosed with lung cancer, reported his cure.

My tumor was about the size of a walnut. I discovered it because I had a horrible cough so my Dr. x-rayed my lungs and found a spot on my lung. He then sent me to have a CT scan and told me it could be cancer. I saw Ralph Cole's banner [for his blog CancerIsOver] on the way home from the doctor that day. I called

Ralph and he gave me a juicer. I juiced for two months and when the doctor x-rayed my lungs after 8 or 9 weeks of juicing the tumor or "spot" on my lungs was gone. The doctor says it was the fact that I quit smoking that made the "spot" or tumor go away. Either way I'm glad it's gone. I told the doctor I juiced and of course medical science doesn't believe in natural remedies so in my doctor's eyes it was the fact that I stopped smoking. I am glad I didn't even have to start any cancer treatments. It is my belief that the carrot juicing took away my tumor.

Cervical and Bladder Cancer

Though Melissa also used radiation, she believes carrot juice cured her cancer. She was diagnosed with cervical cancer in 2012, when she was 24. She declined chemo and tried a variety of natural treatments through November of 2013. She learned in January 2014 that the cancer had spread to her bladder. She had radiation during the month of June 2014, which helped with pain. In July she began juicing five pounds of carrots daily. A CT on August 19, 2014 showed no sign of cancer.

I asked Melissa why she believes that the carrot treatment, rather than the radiation treatment, was responsible for her cure. She wrote me:

"I do believe carrots and nutrition played a more important role to my remission simply because I started feeling better and even my face changed a rosy pink color during the time I was juicing.

I still juice five pounds of carrots every day since it makes me feel so much better and I think a lot more clearly now."

Prostate Cancer

From a review of *Curing Cancer with Carrots* on amazon.com:

My father cured his Stage IV prostate cancer (metastasized to his bones) after the Mayo [Clinic] told him he was too advanced for chemo or radiation. We got him started on carrot juicing (carrots, celery, apple and parsley) 2 -3 times/day. He also used proteolytic enzymes between meals, probiotics, a good multiple/mineral vitamin, Vitamin D and eliminated all sugar, alcohol and animal protein. Within 3 months a follow-up bone scan showed no lesions and his PSA returned to normal. His cancer never did return even though his juicing had become more infrequent and he returned to eating animal products. He eventually died 15 years later (still cancer free) due complications from pulmonary fibrosis.

Glioblastoma Brain Tumor

On May 13, 2013, 72-year-old Alex of New Jersey was diagnosed with an incurable brain tumor, a glioblastoma. Overall, the 1, 5, and 10-year survival rates for patients with this kind of cancer are 33.67%, 4.46%, and 2.7% respectively, making it the most deadly[1] form of all primary brain and central nervous system cancers. Soon after diagnosis, Alex had surgery for it. A few months later, there was a new regrowth of cancer above the spot where the original cancer had been removed. Alex had both radiation and chemotherapy, but doctors had no hope for him and said he would die in a matter of months. With no idea what to do, he and his wife made a spiritual retreat to a European shrine. Another woman on retreat told them about using carrots against cancer. When they returned home, starting May 16, 2014 every day Alex's wife prepared for him the juice from 5 pounds of carrots, 4 apples & 1 stick of celery & a handful of grapes, which produced about 5 glasses of juice. He eliminated red meat and all dairy products from his diet.

His wife reported: "On July 22nd, 2014, an MRI showed not only that the cancer tumor stopped growing but that it had shrunk to just 2 mm. The doctor was very surprised, as they believe there is no cure for glioblastoma cancer. We proved that we could stop it! The doctor said it was a miracle. "Just continue what you've been doing," he said. So we continued with the diet.

"Alex had a new MRI on November 1st, 2014. On a meeting two days later to discuss its findings, the oncologist proclaimed to Alex, "After careful review the MRI shows that you are cancer free!" Can you believe our joy & how wonderful we felt!

Breast Cancer

In 1972 at age 37, Doris of New Canaan, Connecticut received a terminal breast cancer diagnosis. After she had radiation and radical surgery to remove her breast and uterus, her weight dropped from 135 to 80 pounds. She became so weak that she was unable to walk, speak or recognize loved ones. She wouldn't eat, couldn't urinate, and only wanted coffee and pain pills. As her family prepared for her funeral, her husband learned of natural healing techniques developed by the Foundation for Advancement in Cancer Therapy, "He handed me a small juice glass [full of] carrot juice with a straw and he made me drink it... After a month of the juices, I realized what was around me. My eyes got stronger. I was putting on a pound a week. Sleeping pills, tranquilizers, pain pills—in one month's time I was off them all and I was on the carrot juice. ...It took two years before [my] body could handle doing my normal routine, but my cleansing and my diet is the reason I'm here today." [Reported in the New Canaan News, February 18, 2010.]

Rectal Cancer

During the first months of 2014, Rena wrote me from Australia about her husband Nigel's rectal cancer, which his doctors said chemotherapy could not cure.

On January 2, Nigel was diagnosed by PET scan as having rectal cancer with metastases to local lymph nodes and one near the left sternum. We were told it was stage 4. Prognosis: 92% of patients with this stage of cancer die within the first year and 8% make it to two years. The doctors said all they could do was palliative treatment, 6 cycles of chemo. If the tumour shrunk, they would use surgery to remove it.

The 2nd week of January, we started with a very good diet and carrot juice. Nigel drank the juice from five pounds of carrots daily from then to June 2014. Due to family pressure he began chemo, but completed only the first two-week chemo cycle of the recommended six. After getting heart and chest pain at the beginning of the second cycle, he decided no more chemo. He did not want to feel miserable.

May 3, 2014

A new MRI showed no sign of cancer. We talked to the radiation oncologist. Talk about a depressing day. He said although nothing was showing on the MRI - the cancer is going to come back—he requested a PET scan and said even if nothing shows on the PET scan, we should have chemo and radiation as there will be hidden cancer cells that cannot be picked up—I asked, can we not get the cancer surgically removed. He said, "Oh, if you go down that road, you are not trying to cure it." I said, "O.K., say we go down the road you are talking about, which is six months of high dose radiation and chemo, would the cancer come back?" He said he did not know, it may. I looked at Nigel—he looked healthy as ever, no pain, no nothing just orange—I told the radiation oncologist about the carrot juice protocol and he just dismissed me. I asked him what caused the cancer—he said he does not know. How can you cure something when you don't know what caused it?

He even said that the chemo Nigel had does not get rid of the cancer, he said it was to stop growth and delay spread. So I said, "Isn't it amazing that this has regressed and you can't even see it?" DISMISSED again. Aarrrrgh—whilst I type this—Nigel is drinking his carrot juice. I am asking everyone I know to drink freshly squeezed carrot juice whether they have cancer or not!!! My mum and my younger sister have started. My brother in law as well :) To me regression of tumor and resolution of lymph nodes is a good result. Every day he feels good. I guess if we keep the good cells in excellent condition, they can fight the baddy cells.

May 8
Husband had PET scan today, in fact twice, and guess what??? They found nothing. The radiation oncologist was bemused, surprised. Primary tumour cannot be seen, and metastases to distant and local lymph nodes clear. Following the PET, a surgeon gave Nigel a colonoscopy.
It showed no cancer in Nigel's rectum. After the colonoscopy, the surgeon walked into the waiting room and told us, "This is a miracle."
I'm so thrilled. Carrot juices works—one chemo was all he had—carrots, carrots, carrots - he is still carrot juicing daily.

Two doctor friends hearing the story of my own "miracle" responded immediately that I'd been cured by the power of my mind. But I think more than "mind power" is at work. In the cases when carrots have eliminated cancer, the timing is similar—being better in a few days or weeks, and being cured in eight weeks to four months. This time frame is very unlikely to be a coincidence. Especially hopeful for me is that Ralph Cole's experience can definitely be called a cure. He eliminated his tumors in 2006. Eight years later, he's had no further cancer and hasn't resumed juicing carrots. It is too early for me to say that I'm cured like Ralph, but I hope I am. As I write this, I'm two years cancer free.

When many errors in the body's signaling are fixed at once, healthy cells resume their vigilance over rogue cells and eliminate them. So far, carrot juice has stopped many kinds of cancers. Maybe when tumors are too advanced, carrots can't eliminate cancer cells as fast as they proliferate and block essential body functions. If carrots alone don't lead to improvement in two months, a cancer patient should definitely add other approaches.

The speed and ease with which carrots have worked for some of us leads me to visualize some natural cures as fitting particular cancers the way the right key fits a lock. But maybe there are some times when the key doesn't fit the lock, and carrot juice won't work.

Nevertheless, in cases of advanced cancer, when oncologists say that neither radiation nor chemotherapy can cure, people might be better off to abandon those treatments and start using carrots. It's very important not to go halfway with the carrot treatment. Just remember that for a person weighing up to 160 pounds, the cure requires five pounds of carrots daily—more for someone heavier. When processed, five pounds of carrots should produce five cups of juice.

The carrot cure has been proved to make chemotherapy and radiation more effective. However, usually both those treatments reduce appetite and cause nausea, making it difficult to drink much juice.

If you have a very slow-growing cancer, your oncologist might agree to your making a four or six week trial of carrots before chemo or radiation is considered and then order a scan for you. One advantage of that approach is that if your cancer is quickly reduced, you will know that the carrots and not chemo are responsible.

Another is that, if carrots work, you will be spared chemotherapy and radiation, and the high costs and complications that come with them. The disadvantage is that, if carrots don't work, you could suffer tumor growth and delay in starting conventional treatment or turning to other natural alternatives. Weighing these various possibilities is something no one else but you can do.

The Future?

I can envision two futures for nutritional epigenetics in the treatment of cancer. In one, the big drug companies, quite content with the not always successful outcomes of their existing products—which bring far more profits than curing cancer ever could—delay the wide use of natural cancer cures for another thirty years.

In the other, public knowledge of nutritional epigenetics leads to a demand for its development that can't be stopped—revolutionizing cancer treatment and making it faster, pain-free, and affordable for all—a real cure, not a "remission."

If we who get cancer educate ourselves about natural treatments and share the scientific evidence for them, a world of gentle and effective cancer treatments can become a reality. Even better, if we put carrots and other anti-cancer foods into our diets and convince our friends to do the same, we may prevent cancer before it starts, and never have to face its agonizing decisions.

In the cancer adventure with its many bewildering paths, the choices rightly belong to you. If you make the carrot cure part of your journey, I believe that it will help you feel better and may even cure you. By whatever means you choose, I hope you'll soon beat cancer. If carrots help, please share your good news.

Notes

Introduction

1. Anand, Preetha et al. 2008. Cancer is a preventable disease that requires major lifestyle changes." *Pharmaceutical Research* 25.9 (2008): 2097–2116. *PMC.* Web. 14 June 2015.

2. Katz, David L. 2007. Fighting malnutrition among cancer patients. *Medical News Today.* July 19.

3. American Cancer Society. 2014. Cancer facts and figures 2014.

4. Cancer is a preventable disease that requires major lifestyle changes Pharmaceutical Research September 2008 P. Anand, B. Kunnumakara, B. Aggarwal 2008.

One: How the Numbers Melted

1. Royal College of General Practitioners (UK). 2005. Lower gastrointestinal cancer. Referral guidelines for suspected cancer in adults and children. (NICE Clinical Guidelines, No. 27.) 11 Clinical Governance Research and Development Unit (CGRDU), Department of Health Sciences, University of Leicester. June.

2. Le DT, et al. 2015. Mismatch repair deficiency predicts response to pembrolizumab in several cancer types. Abstract LBA100. Presented at: ASCO Annual Meeting; May 29-June

3. Survivorship A to Z. Chemotherapy: Coping with FOLFOX side effects. Accessed June 14, 2015.

Three: The Shooter Misses

1. York University. 2008. Big pharma spends more on advertising than research and development, study finds." *ScienceDaily.* January 7.

Four: Falcarinol and Luteolin

1. Sharma, Krishan Datt et al. 2012. "Chemical composition, functional properties and processing of carrot—a review." *Journal of food science and technology* 49.1 (2012): 22–32. *PMC.* Web. 14 June 2015.

2. Elizabeth Renter. 2013. "Secret weapon" in carrots reduces risk of

cancerous 'full scale tumors' by 1/3. *Natural Society Newsletter*. May 16.

3. Purup, Stig, Larsen, Eric and. Christensen, Lars P. 2009. Differential effects of falcarinol and related aliphatic C_{17}-polyacetylenes on intestinal cell proliferation. *Journal of Agricultural and Food Chemistry* 57.18 (2009): 8290–8296. *PMC*. September 23.

4. Norton, Kyle. 2011. Phytochemicals in foods – 13 health benefits of luteolin. Health Articles. December 31.

5. Miean KH1, Mohamed S. 2001. Flavonoid (myricetin, quercetin, kaempferol, luteolin, and apigenin) content of edible tropical plants. *J Agric Food Chem*. 49(6):3106-12. June.

6. Liu RH[1]. 2004. Potential synergy of phytochemicals in cancer prevention: mechanism of action. *J Nutr.* 134(12 Suppl):3479S-3485S. December.

Five: Juicing Carrots

1 Differential Effects of Falcarinol and Related Aliphatic C17-Polyacetylenes on Intestinal Cell Proliferation J Agric Food Chem. 2009 Sep 23 Purup, Larsen, Christensen. 2009.

2. Durenberger, Caleb. 2014. Is too much betacarotene bad for you? Livestrong.com. February 2.

3. Yang, CS. Suh N, Kong, AN. 2012. Does vitamin E prevent or promote cancer? *Cancer Prevention Research*, 5(5):701-5. doi: 10.1158/1940-6207.CAPR-12-0045. May.

4. Chris Kresser. 2012. The little known (but crucial) difference between folate and folic acid. Let's Take Back Your Health. March 9.

Six: Treating the Community of Cells

1. Wigle, Dennis, and Igor Jurisica, Igor. 2007. Cancer as a system failure. *Cancer Informatics* 5 (2007): 10–18. Print.

2. Wilde, Monica. 2012 Plant nutrients and the genes that suppress the spread of cancer. Napiers the Herbalists. Sept. 26.

3. McKie, Robin. 2013. Why do identical twins end up having such different lives? *The Guardian*. June 2.

4. Sung, Bokyung et al. 2012. Cancer cell signaling pathways targeted by spice-derived nutraceuticals." *Nutrition and cancer* 64.2 (2012): 173–197.

5. 2013. Phytochemicals: the cancer fighters in the foods we eat. American Institute for Cancer Research. April 10.

6. Li, William. 2010. Can we eat to starve cancer? TED talk. February.

7. Venter, Craig. 2008. Genes have very little impact on life outcomes. *India Today*. March 31.

8. 2012. Structural biochemistry/cell signaling pathways/problems in signaling that cause cancer. Wikibooks. July 12.

9. Link A1, Balaguer F, Goel A. 2010. Cancer chemoprevention by dietary polyphenols: promising role for epigenetics. *Biochem Pharmacol.* 80(12):1771-92. doi: 10.1016/j.bcp.2010.06.036. December 15.

10. Rakoff-Nahoum, Seth. 2006. Why cancer and Inflammation? *The Yale Journal of Biology and Medicine* 79.3-4 (2006): 123–130. December.

Seven: Apoptosis and Necrosis

1. Geever, John. 2012. Tumor lysis syndrome common in some cancers. *MedPage Today*. Dec. 11.

2. 2000. Favourable and unfavourable effects on long-term survival of radiotherapy for early breast cancer: an overview of the randomised trials. Early Breast Cancer Trialists' Collaborative Group. Lancet. 355(9217):1757-70.. May 20.

3. 2006. Common cancer treatments toxic to healthy brain cells. Rochester scientists isolate source of 'chemo brain.' University of Rochester Medical Center Newsroom. Nov. 30.

4. Sherry Baker. 2010. Cancer cells killed by chemotherapy may cause cancer to spread. *Natural News*. June 22.

5. Byrne, Michael. 2014. Zombie Cancer Cells Are a Problem. *Motherboard*. April 6.

Eight: Caution and Chemotherapy

1. Audrey, Suzanne et al. 2008. What oncologists tell patients about survival benefits of palliative chemotherapy and implications for informed consent: qualitative study." *BM: British Medical Journal* 337 (2008): a752. July 31.

2. Boseley, Sarah. 2008. Questions raised over chemotherapy for late-stage cancer. *The Guardian.* November 12.

3. Chen, Pauline W. 2012. Poor pain control for cancer patients. *New York Times.* Sept. 20.

4. Ji, Sayer. 2012. Chemo and radiation can make cancer more malignant. Green Med Info. July 31.

5. Cancer multidrug resistance. 2000. *Nature Biotechnology* 18, IT18 - IT20.

6. Foote, MaryAnn. 1998. The importance of planned dose of chemotherapy on time: do we need to change our clinical practice? *The Oncologist.* vol. 3 no. 5 365-368. October.

7. Begg, Colin B. and Schrag, Deborah. 2002. Attribution of deaths following cancer treatment. *Journal of the National Cancer Institute. 94 (14): 1044-1045.*

8. Angell, Marcia. 2004. The Truth About the Drug Companies: How They Deceive Us and What to Do About It, New York: Random House. p. 95.

9. Angell, Marcia. 2009. Drug companies and doctors: a story of corruption. *New York Review of Books.* January 15.

Nine: Carrot Liberation

1. Kolata, Gina and Pollack, Andrew. 2008. Costly cancer drug offers hope but also a dilemma. *New York Times.* July 6.

2. Goodman, Brenda. 2011. Cancer drug Avastin linked to death risk. Web MD. News Archive. February 1.

3. Harvard Heart Letter. 2012. Cancer treatments may harm the heart. Doctors strive to prevent the cure for one disease from causing another. August 1.

4. Bagli E[1], Stefaniotou M, Morbidelli L, Ziche M, Psillas K, Murphy C, Fotsis T. 2004. Luteolin inhibits vascular endothelial growth factor-induced angiogenesis; inhibition of endothelial cell survival and proliferation by targeting phosphatidylinositol 3'-kinase activity. *Cancer Research.* November 1.

5. Gonzalez-Angulo, A.M., Morales-Vasquez, F., Hortobagyi, G.M. 2007. Overview of resistance to systemic therapy in patients with breast cancer. *Advances in Experimental Medicine and Biology* 608:1-22.

6. McEwen, Bruce S. 2003. Estrogen effects on the brain: much more than sex. *Karger Gazette* No. 66. 608:1-22.

7. Eberling, J.L., Wu, C., Tong-Turnbeaugh, R., Jagust, WJ. 2004. Estrogen- and tamoxifen-associated effects on brain structure and function. Neuroimage 21(1):364-71. January.

8. Gordon, Serena. 2013. Tamoxifen's mental side effects are real: study. Wed MD News Archive. September 17.

9. 2009. Long-term tamoxifen use increases risk of an aggressive, hard to treat type of second breast cancer. *Science Daily.* August.10.

10. Zivian, Marilyn T. and Salgado. Brenda. 2008. Side effects revisited: women's experiences with aromatase inhibitors. Breast Cancer Action. June.SIDE EFFECTS.

11. 2012. Vegetable pigment luteolin suppresses estrogen production. Foodforbreastcancer.com. August 5.

Ten: Puzzles of Profitability

1. Oncologist Salary. Health Care Salaries. http://www.healthcare-salaries.com/physicians/oncologist-salary.

2. Gatesman, Mandy L. and Smith, Thomas J. 2011. The shortage of essential chemotherapy drugs in the United States. N Engl J Med 2011; 365:1653-1655. November 3: 10.1056/NEJMp1109772

3. E. Haavi Morreim, E. Haavi. Prescribing Under the Influence. Markkula Center for Applied Ethics, Santa Clara University.

4. Lee, John R, Zava, David and Hopkins, Virginia. 2002. "The history and politics of the breast cancer industry; Why we just can't

seem to prevent or cure breast cancer." In *How hormone balance can help save your life*, New York, Warner Books.

Eleven: Making Decisions

1. http://www.polst.org/

2. http://theconversationproject.org/

3. Julie Creswell and Reed Abelson. 2014. Hospital Chain Said to Scheme to Inflate Bills. nytimes.com. January 23

4. 2007. Fighting malnutrition among cancer patients. *Medical News Today*. July 19.

5. King, N.B. and Fraser, V. 2013. Untreated pain, narcotics regulation, and global health ideologies. *PLoS Med*. April 2.

6. Welch, H. Gilbert, Albertson, Peter C., Nease, Robert F., Bubolz, Thomas A., and Wasson, John H. 1996. Estimating treatment benefits for the elderly: the effect of competing risks. *Annals of Internal Medicine* Vol 123 No. 6. March 15.

7. 2013. Death by for-profit health care. *Strike Debt!* March 26.

8. Rauch, Jonathan. 2013. How not to die: Angelo Volandes's low-tech, high-empathy plan to revolutionize end-of-life care. *The Atlantic*. May 2013.

9. 2012. Dr. Otis Brawley: 'The system really is not failing … Failure Is The System'. *Kaiser Health News*. May 1.

10. Arnst, Catherine. 2009. Study Links Medical Costs and Personal Bankruptcy. *Business Week*. June 4.

11. Robertson, Christopher T., Egelhof, Richard, and Hoke, Michael. 2008. Get sick, get out: the medical causes of home foreclosures. *Health Matrix* 18 (2008): 65-105.

12. Paddock, Catharine. 2013. Stress fuels cancer spread by triggering master gene. *Medical News Today*. August 27.

13. Neergaard, Lauran. 2013. Report: boomers face crisis in cancer

care. *USA Today*. September 10.

14. 2013. Chemotherapy-Related Hospitalizations Common in Palliative Care. American Society of Clinical Oncology. November 1.

15. Span, Paula. 2012. End-of-life care: Misunderstanding chemo. *New York Times*. November 12.

16. Brink, Susan. 2013. Weighing over-treatment vs. ending treatment: When it comes to cancer, do last-ditch treatment efforts do more harm than good? *U.S. News and World Report Health*. October 11.

17. NPR Staff. 2012. 'Best care': we make death harder than it has to be. National Public Radio Interview. March 26.

18. Brink, Susan. 2013. Weighing Over-Treatment vs. Ending Treatment. usnews.com.: October 11.

19. CTV. 2013. Many terminal cancer patients want more end-of-life options: study. CTV News. May 1.

20. 2014. Study shows more hospital deaths and invasive care for dying cancer patients who receive chemotherapy. Dana Farber Cancer Institute. March 4.

21. Harrington, Sarah Elizabeth and Smith, Thomas J. 2011. The role of chemotherapy at the end of life: When Is enough, enough? Journal of the American Medical Association. June 11.

Twelve: Cures with Carrots

1. Tocagen Brain Cancer Statistics.
www.tocagen.com/programs/brain-cancer-statistics/

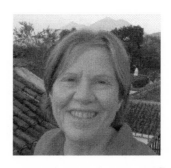

The author of internationally acclaimed children's books, Ann Cameron grew up in in Rice Lake, Wisconsin, U.S.A. She is an honors graduate of Harvard University, where she was awarded the James Bryant Conant Prize for science writing. She spends most of the year in Panajachel, Guatemala, where she and her late husband, Bill, rebuilt the local library with 13,000 donated books. It has been used as a model throughout the country. She continues to write surrounded by palm trees, flowers and butterflies near the shores of Lake Atitlán.

You may contact me at curingcancerwithcarrots@hotmail.com

Made in the USA
Las Vegas, NV
16 November 2020